Management of stable angina

Edited by

David de Bono
Professor of Cardiology, University of Leicester

Anthony Hopkins
Director, Research Unit, Royal College of Physicians

1994

ROYAL COLLEGE OF PHYSICIANS OF LONDON

BRITISH CARDIAC SOCIETY

Royal College of Physicians of London
11 St Andrews Place, London NW1 4LE

Registered Charity No. 210508

Copyright © 1994 Royal College of Physicians of London
ISBN 1 873240 65 1

Typeset by Dan-Set Graphics, Telford, Shropshire
Printed in Great Britain by Cathedral Print Services Ltd, Salisbury

Editors' introduction

David de Bono
Professor of Cardiology, University of Leicester
Anthony Hopkins
Director, Research Unit, Royal College of Physicians

The origin of this book was a workshop set up under the auspices of the Joint Audit Committee of the British Cardiac Society and the Royal College of Physicians of London to advise on standards of care for the management of patients presenting with the symptoms of angina pectoris, and to identify ways of auditing such care. The chapters of the book were originally presented as working papers for discussion. They have been edited so as to provide a structured approach to the problem.

The first chapter summarises current concepts in the pathology and physiology of coronary heart disease. The second and third chapters, from Professor David Wood and Professor John Hampton, consider the incidence and prevalence of angina pectoris in the community, and discuss the methodological techniques and problems of measurement. Professor Wood's chapter concentrates on the assessment of incidence, ie the number of new cases presenting in a defined population over a given period of time, whereas Professor Hampton's chapter is more concerned with prevalence, ie the total number of angina cases, new and continuing, in the community. An important point in both chapters is that angina, a symptom, is a surrogate marker for the prevalence of ischaemic heart disease in the underlying community. Community variations in angina probably reflect variations in the incidence of coronary heart disease. Angina also identifies a high risk group of patients with coronary heart disease in terms of complications, morbidity and mortality. However, it should be remembered that most patients presenting with myocardial infarction, particularly in younger age groups, come from the population with clinically silent coronary disease, who have never had warning angina.

It emerges clearly from Chapters 2 and 3 that the vast majority of patients with angina are looked after by general practitioners, and that general practitioners have an important function as gatekeepers to the scarcer and more expensive resources offered by hospital investigation. In Chapter 4, Dr John Inman examines the role of general practitioners, and discusses the factors that lead to hospital referral. An important distinction is made between patients with classical symptoms of angina, in whom referral is made either for risk assessment or for consideration of non-pharmacological treatment, and the group of patients in whom the clinical diagnosis is uncertain, when the referral is made for clarification of diagnosis.

This theme is taken up in Chapter 5 by Dr John Irving, who considers the role of the district hospital cardiologist or physician with special training and experience in cardiology in assessing and managing patients referred by the general practitioner. A structured assessment scheme is proposed, with equal emphasis on clinical assessment and exercise electrocardiography. The scope and limitations of exercise electrocardiography are critically discussed.

In the following chapters, Dr Raphael Balcon and Dr Simon Davies discuss the role of coronary angiography in diagnosis, risk stratification, and assessment for intervention, and one of us (D de B) outlines the expected outcomes from interventions such as angioplasty and coronary bypass grafting. Again a clear distinction is made between the circumstances in which intervention is performed to improve survival and those in which it is performed with the primary purpose of improving symptoms.

In the subsequent chapters, an attempt is made to relate the practice of patient care to the framework of investigation already presented, and to identify the problems faced by current practice in meeting these standards. Dr John Birkhead gives a personal account of the handling of patients with suspected angina in a district general hospital, he and Dr Dudley Pennell and Dr Richard Underwood consider the role of nuclear cardiology in the investigation of patients with angina, and Dr Michael Joy discusses the needs of a district hospital for referral to specialist cardiac centres. One of us (D de B) describes what happens to patients in such centres. Dr David Gray then discusses the results of studies that attempted to evaluate variations in patient management and practice in different specialist cardiac centres within the same health region.

In the final chapters, Dr Birkhead and Dr Peter Wilkinson discuss a possible framework for audit in cardiological practice, with emphasis on the need for defining minimal data sets and on the need for a continuous audit process. The final chapter summarises the data and concepts presented earlier, and also suggests minimum data sets and information requirement for the audit of angina care at primary, secondary and tertiary care levels.

Purchasers of health care, both fundholding general practitioners and district health authorities, will be specifying with
tighter focus the services that they expect their patients to receive.
We believe that they will find this book useful. Cardiologists, general practitioners and those in training will also find in these pages
useful reviews of the effectiveness of their practice.

Contributors

Raphael Balcon, *Consultant Cardiologist, The London Chest Hospital, Bonner Road, London E2 9JX·*

John S Birkhead, *Consultant Physician, Northampton General Hospital, Northampton NN1 5BD*

Simon Davies *(Rapporteur), formerly Senior Registrar in Cardiology, The London Chest Hospital, Bonner Road, London E2 9JX; now Consultant Cardiologist, Royal Brompton National Heart and Lung Hospital, Sydney Street, London SW3 6NP*

David P de Bono, *Professsor of Cardiology, University of Leicester, Glenfield Hospital NHS Trust, Groby Road, Leicester LE3 9QP*

David Gray, *Senior Lecturer in Medicine, Department of Medicine, University Hospital, Queen's Medical Centre, Nottingham NG7 2UH*

John R Hampton, *Professor of Cardiology, Department of Medicine, University Hospital, Queen's Medical Centre, Nottingham NG7 2UH*

John K Inman, *General Practitioner, The Health Centre, Melton Road, Syston, Leicester LE7 8EQ*

John B Irving, *Consultant Physician, St John's Hospital at Howden, Howden Road West, Livingston, West Lothian EH54 6PP*

Michael D Joy, *Consultant Physician and Cardiologist, St Peter's Hospital, Chertsey, Surrey KT16 0PZ*

Dudley J Pennell, *Senior Lecturer in Cardiac Imaging, Magnetic Resonance Unit, Royal Brompton National Heart and Lung Hospital, Sydney Street, London SW3 6NP*

S Richard Underwood, *Senior Lecturer in Cardiac Imaging, Magnetic Resonance Unit, Royal Brompton National Heart and Lung Hospital, Sydney Street, London SW3 6NP*

Peter R Wilkinson, *Consultant Physician, Ashford Hospital, London Road, Ashford, Middlesex TW15 3AA*

David Wood, *Honorary Consultant Cardiologist, National Heart and Lung Institute, Dovehouse Street, London SW3 6LY*

Other participants at the workshop

Stuart Cobbe, *Walton Professor of Medical Cardiology, Royal Infirmary, Glasgow*

Kim Fox, *Consultant Cardiologist, Royal Brompton National Heart and Lung Hospital, London*

Anthony Hopkins, *Director, Research Unit, Royal College of Physicians, London*

Cyril R Nyman, *Consultant Physician in Cardio-Respiratory Medicine, Pilgrim Hospital, Boston, Lincolnshire*

Shakeel Qureshi, *Consultant Paediatric Cardiologist, Guy's Hospital, London*

Josie Thomas, *Senior Chief Technician, Department of Cardiology, University of Leicester School of Medicine, Glenfield General Hospital, Leicester*

Robert West, *Department of Epidemiology, University of Wales College of Medicine, Cardiff*

Richard Wray, *Consultant Physician (Cardiology), Conquest Hospital, St Leonards on Sea, East Sussex*

Acknowledgements

The Royal College of Physicians is grateful to the Department of Health for a contribution to the running costs of the workshop. Administrative asssistance and secretarial support to the workshop were provided by Janice Bowman, Barbara Durr and Fiona Shipley. The Research Unit of the College is supported by grants from the Wolfson and Welton Foundations, other charitable donations, and by the Department of Health.

Contents

1 | Pathophysiology of ischaemic heart disease

David de Bono
Professor of Cardiology, University of Leicester

Rational policies for the management of suspected ischaemic heart disease must be based on a knowledge of the underlying pathophysiology and natural history. For the purposes of this chapter, ischaemic heart disease will be regarded as virtually synonymous with atheromatous coronary artery disease.

Pathology

The characteristic lesions of atheromatous coronary disease have been well described in several standard texts and reviews.[1,2] The presence of an unobstructed lumen as seen on angiography during life does not necessarily exclude atheromatous disease in the vessel wall.

There is a biological continuum between patients with isolated coronary stenoses and those in whom virtually the entire coronary tree is affected by advanced atheromatous disease. In general, patients with isolated lesions tend to be younger, and in the United Kingdom they are often smokers with isolated hypercholesterolaemia. Diffuse disease is more common in older patients, diabetics, and patients of South Asian origin. Coronary disease assessed at postmortem tends to be more extensive than that apparent on angiography during life.

Progression of coronary lesions

It is clear from serial angiographic studies that individual coronary lesions evolve or progress at very different rates. Thus an apparently unaffected segment of the coronary tree may develop a severe stenosis over a time scale of a few weeks or months, while an established stenosis in an adjacent section remains unaltered.[3] Rapid progression of a lesion may be due to the formation and subsequent organisation of thrombus on a lesion where a thrombogenic surface has been exposed by cracking or by endothelial damage. Progression may also be due to the sudden influx of macrophages into a fatty lesion as a variety of inflammatory reaction to the presence of partially oxidised lipids. If flow in a coronary artery, particularly the right coronary artery, is reduced by a severe stenosis, the diameter of the vessel, both proximal and distal to the stenosis, sometimes diminishes rapidly over a time course of a few months. This is presumably a consequence of the normal physiological relationship between blood flow velocity and vessel diameter.

Coronary occlusion

The commonest mechanism for the complete occlusion of a coronary artery is thrombosis on the basis of a cracked or ruptured atheromatous plaque.[4,5] Factors that determine whether fissuring and thrombosis occur include the morphology of the plaque[6] and its lipid and macrophage content.[7] Not only does thrombotic coronary occlusion prevent forward flow at the site of the blockage, but there is increasing evidence that it inhibits retrograde flow through any collateral circulation by the vasoactive effects of thrombin and of products of platelet activation released from the clot. The usual consequence of thrombotic coronary occlusion in a vessel that had previously carried substantial blood flow is therefore myocardial infarction. Silent coronary occlusion without myocardial infarction is more likely to occur if the process of occlusion is very gradual. This gives time for an adequate collateral circulation to develop, and since the final occluding thrombus is likely to be extremely small it will produce little in the way of vasoactive substances to impede the collateral circulation. Many thrombotic coronary occlusions subsequently recanalise under the influence of fibrinolytic agents released from the adjacent arterial wall.[8] This recanalisation is most likely to occur in relatively large vessels where the obstruction of the lumen by atheromatous plaque, as opposed to thrombus, is incomplete. The time course of recanalisation is however usually too slow to preserve the viability of distal myocardium.

Collateral circulation. During coronary angioplasty, when a vessel is transiently occluded by balloon inflation, collateral flow from the contralateral coronary artery can be demonstrated in up to 50% of cases. Conversely, after abrupt coronary occlusion by thrombosis, collateral flow can be demonstrated angiographically in only 5% of patients at one hour, increasing to 25% at 24 and 50% at 48 hours. The possible negative effects of thrombus on collateral flow have been discussed above. There is some evidence that collateral circulation can be improved by physical exercise, and that this can be inhibited by beta-adrenoceptor blocking drugs.

Association of coronary artery disease and myocardial disease

In patients with isolated non-occlusive coronary stenoses, the myocardium downstream is usually macroscopically normal. Careful microscopic examination, particularly in patients who die suddenly or who have previously had unstable angina, sometimes reveals the presence of platelet microemboli. Myocardial infarction causes necrosis of muscle supplied by the blocked vessel, although the extreme endocardial and epicardial layers are usually spared. If the patient survives, the necrotic myocardium is replaced by fibrous scar tissue. There is some evidence that the subsequent expansion of the scar tissue to form a ventricular aneurysm is diminished by previous thrombolytic therapy, which may improve the survival of epicardial muscle even though there is no apparent effect on ventricular ejection fraction, and also by angiotensin converting enzyme inhibitors.

In patients with extensive and severe coronary artery disease there is frequently evidence of myocardial scarring both on gross and on microscopic examination, whether or not the patient had previously complained of the clinical features of myocardial infarction. Extensive myocardial scarring may be associated with progressive biventricular dilatation and ultimately death from pump failure.

Physiology of ischaemic heart disease

Exercise in a patient with an isolated fairly severe coronary stenosis is associated with impaired contractility in the area of myocardium supplied by that vessel, as detected by radionuclide studies, electrocardiographic (ECG) changes of myocardial ischaemia, and chest pain, usually in that order. These changes are reversed when exercise ceases. The clinical diagnosis of angina is based on the occurrence of characteristic chest pain on exertion which is relieved by rest. The electrocardiographic changes form the basis for the detection and confirmation of ischaemic heart disease by exercise testing and/or ambulatory ECG monitoring (Chapter 5). Because the ECG changes are frequently a more sensitive indicator of ischaemia than the patient's perception of chest pain, ambulatory ECG monitoring frequently reveals episodes of 'silent ischaemia', and the patient may not be aware that he or she is suffering from ischaemic heart disease. The parallel response of silent ischaemia and of perceived angina to medication suggests that their mechanism is identical.[9]

The severity of anginal symptoms as reported by the patient is poorly correlated with either the extent or the number of coronary stenoses as determined by angiography or by post mortem studies. There are several reasons for this poor correlation. The haemodynamic obstruction caused by coronary stenosis is a non-linear function of vessel diameter at the site of stenosis, so stenoses of less than 70% of the lumen diameter cause significant coronary obstruction only at extreme exercise levels. Moreover, simple measurement of vessel diameter is a very inadequate way of expressing the haemodynamic obstruction which may be due to tandem lesions extending over a considerable length of the coronary artery. In patients with multiple stenoses, but without coronary obstruction, exercise tolerance is probably limited by the single vessel or lesion with the greatest degree of functional haemodynamic obstruction.

Although pain is an insensitive index of the mass of ischaemic myocardium, this will be more realistically mirrored by functional impairment, as indicated by a fall in global ejection fraction during exercise and, in severe cases, by a fall in blood pressure and the development of presyncopal symptoms as exercise proceeds.

Modes of death in ischaemic heart disease

A high proportion of sudden deaths in patients with ischaemic heart disease are associated with acute thrombotic coronary occlusion.[10] The commonest cause of death associated with acute coronary obstruction is acute ventricular fibrillation. This is relatively independent of the area of myocardium at risk, and patients resuscitated from acute ventricular fibrillation do not have a worse long-term ventricular function or a worse long-term prognosis. A proportion of patients develop late ventricular arrhythmias, usually a monomorphic ventricular tachycardia, two to three days after myocardial infarction. This is associated with extensive ventricular damage, and usually with a poor long-term prognosis. It is thought that extensive damage and scarring in the ventricle create a substrate for unstable re-entry circuits.

Patients suffering from severe myocardial ischaemia may develop ventricular arrhythmias, including ventricular fibrillation, during the course of a severe anginal attack. The mechanism presumably involves a combination of the immediate effects of myocardial ischaemia and of raised catecholamine levels. It is likely, though not proven, that this risk is diminished considerably with the widespread use of beta-adrenoceptor blockers. Patients with severe impairment of ventricular function as a consequence of chronic ischaemic heart disease are also prone to sudden death as a result of ventricular arrhythmias. In this instance, the likely mechanism is disruption of the normal intraventricular conduction pathways and homogeneity of excitation and repolarisation, coupled with high catecholamine levels which invariably accompany chronic cardiac failure.

Patients may also die as a result of pump failure in end-stage coronary heart disease.

Aetiology of coronary artery disease

Coronary artery disease has been epitomised as a response to a chronic series of insults delivered to the vessel wall and its endothelial lining. The main risk factors, for which a causative role can definitely be accepted, are listed in Table 1.

Table 1. Risk factors for atheromatous coronary disease.

Major factors	*Possible factors*
Smoking	Hyperfibrinogenaemia
Hypercholesterolaemia	Increased clotting factor VII
Diabetes	Hypertriglyceridaemia (especially for
Hypertension	myocardial infarction)
	Deficient fibrinolysis

Smoking

Smoking is accepted as a major risk factor by epidemiological association, but the precise mechanisms are uncertain. Smoking is known to increase vascular reactivity and, in some patients, susceptibility to vascular spasm, probably mediated by nicotine. Smoking is known to cause endothelial damage, perhaps mediated by oxygen free-radicals, and it may increase oxidation of vessel wall lipids. Smoking is associated with increased plasma fibrinogen concentration and with diminished activity of plasma free-radical scavengers (some of which may be due to a reduced dietary intake).

Hyperlipidaemia

Coronary atheroma is associated with raised total cholesterol and a low ratio of total cholesterol to HDL cholesterol. The relationship is particularly striking in patients with familial hypercholesterolaemia, and appears to be independent of the mechanism of hypercholesterolaemia. Hypertriglyceridaemia seems to be more closely associated with the risk of myocardial infarction than with coronary atheroma, possibly because it affects blood coagulation and thrombolysis.

Diabetes

Diabetes mellitus, whether insulin requiring or non-insulin dependent, is associated with precocious and extensive coronary artery disease. Hyperinsulinaemic states, particularly those associated with obesity and mild hypertension, are also associated with coronary disease. This may be mediated partly through abnormalities in lipid metabolism but also through abnormalities in the matrix of the vessel wall.

Hypertension

Hypertension is strongly associated with an increased risk of ischaemic heart disease and cardiac events. Early trials failed to show an impact of antihypertensive treatment on coronary events but this may have been an artefact of trial design. Recent studies on hypertension in the elderly have clearly shown that control of hypertension reduces the risk of myocardial infarction and cardiac death.

Conclusion

The pathophysiology of ischaemic heart disease is largely that of atheromatous coronary artery disease and its thrombotic complications. The natural history of atheromatous coronary disease is one of gradual background progression, interspersed with episodes of rapid progression as a result of acute changes within individual lesions. The total atheromatous burden of the coronary circulation tends to represent an integration over time of both genetic susceptibility and exposure to risk factors. In contrast, a patient's symptoms often reflect acute changes in a single critical lesion.

The coronary circulation has considerable capacity for biological adaptation. In contrast, myocardial damage, once it has occurred, tends to be permanent.

Prevention of death from ischaemic heart disease requires both the protection of the heart from sudden severe ischaemia and the prevention of extensive ventricular damage.

References

1. Fuster V, Badimon L, Badimon J, Chesebro J. Mechanisms of disease: the pathogenesis of coronary artery disease and the acute coronary syndromes. I. *New England Journal of Medicine* 1992; **326**: 242–50.
2. Fuster V, Badimon L, Badimon J, Chesebro J. Mechanisms of disease: the pathogenesis of coronary artery disease and the acute coronary syndromes. II. *New England Journal of Medicine* 1992; **326**: 310–8.
3. Singh RN. Progression of coronary atherosclerosis: clues to pathogenesis from serial coronary arteriography. *British Heart Journal* 1984; **32**: 451–61.
4. Davies MJ, Thomas AC. Plaque fissuring: the cause of acute myocardial infarction, sudden ischaemic death and crescendo angina. *British Heart Journal* 1985; **53**: 63–73.
5. Falk E. Unstable angina with fatal outcome: dynamic coronary thrombosis leading to infarction and/or sudden death. *Circulation* 1985; **71**: 699–708.
6. Richardson P, Davies M, Born G. Influence of plaque configuration and stress distribution on fissuring of coronary atherosclerotic plaques. *Lancet* 1989; **ii**: 941–4.
7. Davies MJ, Richardson PD, Woolf N, Katz DR, Mann J. Risk of thrombosis in human atherosclerotic plaques: role of extracellular lipid, macrophage, and smooth muscle content. *British Heart Journal* 1993; **69**: 377–81.
8. Underwood M, de Bono DP. Increased fibrinolytic activity in the intima of atheromatous coronary arteries: protection at a price? *Cardiovascular Research* 1993; **27**: 882–5.
9. Mulcahy D, Parameshwar J, Holdright D, Wright C, Sparrow J, Sultan G, Fox KM. Value of ambulatory ST segment monitoring in patients with chronic stable angina: does measurement of the 'total ischaemic burden' assist with management? *British Heart Journal* 1992; **67**: 47–52.
10. Davies MJ, Thomas A. Thrombosis and acute coronary artery lesions in sudden cardiac ischaemic death. *New England Journal of Medicine* 1984; **310**: 1137–40.

2 | Incidence and prognosis of angina

David Wood
Honorary Consultant Cardiologist,
National Heart and Lung Institute, London

The frequency of angina pectoris, its clinical course and its prognosis should be studied in the general population because selected hospital cases are biased in terms of their clinical characteristics and prognosis. Traditionally population surveys of angina have been the province of epidemiologists using simple, cheap, valid and reproducible measures, such as the WHO chest pain questionnaire,[1] to identify cases and measure prognosis. Prevalence of angina is the measure most commonly reported,[2] but as it reflects both incidence and survival it is the least valuable. Only incident cases with follow-up will give a complete clinical picture of this disease in the population. Whilst these surveys give an accurate population measure of disease frequency, this is at the expense of individual misclassification, unlike clinical practice where correct diagnosis is of paramount importance. A further limitation of this epidemiological approach is the absence of any cardiovascular investigation, other than a resting ECG, in assessing prognosis; therefore, not unexpectedly, the predictive value of these simple tests for myocardial ischaemia, infarction and cardiac death is weak.[3] A population survey of angina ideally should identify incident cases, diagnosed individually, who can be clinically assessed with appropriate cardiological investigations and followed up for prognosis.

Population studies of angina

Five prospective population studies of incident angina have been reported,[4-8] one in America, one in Israel, and three in the UK (Edinburgh, London, and our own survey in Southampton) (Table 1). Three studies (Framingham, Edinburgh, Southampton) were based on general population samples, one on an occupational cohort of civil servants, and one on the population of a single general practitioner. Men only were studied in Edinburgh and Israel but the other studies included men and women. With the exception of Fry's survey of his own general practice in London,

David Wood

Table 1. Incidence and prognosis of angina pectoris in population surveys.

Study	Population	Diagnosis	Investigations	Incidence	Prognosis
Kannel 1972 (Ref. 4)	Healthy men and women, 30–62 yrs, Framingham, Massachusetts, USA, interviewed at biennial examinations	Clinical; 3 physicians (structured questionnaire)	ECG, CXR	Age-specific incidence rates/ 1,000/annum in men (and women) ranged from about 3% (<1%) for 40–44 yrs to 11% (8%) for 60–64 yrs	Over 14-year follow-up 48% (57/119) of men and 25% (27/110) of women with angina had another manifestation of CHD (MI and/or death) of whom 58% (31/57) men and 52% (14/27) women died in total. Remission of new angina in 32% of men and 44% of women for at least 2 years
Medalie 1976 (Ref. 10)	Healthy male civil service and municipal employees, ≥40 yrs; Israeli ischaemic heart disease study	Clinical; several physicians (structured questionnaire)	ECG	Age-adjusted incidence rate of new angina in men 5.7/1,000/annum	Of 256 men with definite new angina, 85% alive and well at 5 yrs, 7% suffered MI, 3% died, the rest (5%) unreported

	Population	Method of diagnosis	Investigations	Incidence	Outcome
Fry 1976 (Ref. 6)	Healthy men and women, >40 yrs, in one general practice population of about 2,755	Clinical; 1 GP		Crude incidence rate of angina, including angina in those with MI (23% of all cases) in adults >40 yrs 5/1,000/annum (56% >60 yrs at time of diagnosis)	Over 20-year follow-up 50% (134/268) patients died, three quarters from cardiovascular cause (annual mortality 4.6%), 7% (20/263) developed complications (MI and cardiac failure). In 25% (67/268) angina persisted; in 18% (47/268) it resolved
Duncan 1976 (Ref. 7)	Men <70 yrs with chest pain referred from 71 selected GPs with population of 28,400 men, 35–69 yrs	Clinical; 1 cardiologist taking account of all investigations	ECG, CXR, enzymes. When diagnosis in doubt, exercise test performed	Crude incidence rate for new angina in men (10% had history of MI) 1.8/1,000/annum	14% (18/129) of new angina cases developed cardiac complications (MI and death) over 6 months from time of presentation
Gandhi 1992 (Ref. 8)	Men and women <70 yrs with new chest pain referred from random sample of 117 GPs with population of 191,677	Clinical; 1 cardiologist (structured questionnaire)	ECG, CXR, exercise test and 24 h ambulatory ECG tape	Crude incidence rate (95% CI) for new angina 0.83 (0.66, 1.0)/1,000/annum	

where more than 20% of cases were aged over 70 years at the time of diagnosis, the other studies were restricted to working adults below this age.

In all these studies the diagnosis of angina was made by at least one physician taking the history, and a standardised questionnaire was often used. In Framingham two physicians interviewed all suspected cases of angina and a third made the final decision without knowledge of the patient's risk factors for coronary heart disease (CHD). In all but one of these surveys the diagnosis was solely historical and no account was taken of other investigations, but the cardiologist in Edinburgh took into account the results of a resting ECG and chest X-ray (and in doubtful cases an exercise test as well) when making the diagnosis. Fry did not routinely employ further investigations. All other studies included a resting ECG, and in some cases a chest X-ray and exercise test, but our Southampton survey is the only one systematically to exercise all new patients with angina. Whilst all these surveys were based primarily on new cases of angina, with no past history of CHD, in Framingham, Edinburgh and London patients with angina who had other manifestations of CHD were included. The prognosis of angina is reported by four of these studies (Framingham, Edinburgh, Israel and London) in relation to serious cardiac complications including death.

Framingham heart study

The Framingham heart study was the first prospective survey of incident angina in men and women in one population, a sample of residents in Framingham, Massachusetts.[4] More than 5,000 healthy men and women (30–62 years) were invited to have a biennial examination at which a physician asked about chest discomfort, using a standardised questionnaire. A patient suspected to have angina pectoris was then independently interviewed by a second physician and the two physicians had to agree that the condition was present. A review committee consisting of three physicians, unaware of the patient's cardiovascular risk profile, made the final decision. Electrocardiographic abnormalities, either at rest or with exertion, were not required for the diagnosis. Cases with an underlying cardiac cause, eg aortic valve disease, were excluded.

Symptoms of angina were common as a first clinical manifestation of CHD in both men and women in this study. Angina occurred in 37% of men with CHD and in 61% of women. Although a higher proportion of women presented in this way, the age-specific annual incidence rate for angina was consistently higher in men, the gap between the sexes narrowing with advancing age. The estimated age-specific incidence rates per 1,000 per annum for men and women ranged from about 3% and <1% in those aged 40–44 years to 11% and 8% in those aged 60–64 years. When patients presented with angina without any other manifestation of CHD (acute ischaemia, infarction or death) between biennial examinations, ie 'uncomplicated angina', this was about as frequent in women as in men.

Over a 14-year follow-up, 48% (57/119) of men and 25% (27/110) of women with angina had a more serious manifestation of CHD (myocardial infarction and/or death), demonstrating a poorer prognosis for men. The probability of a coronary attack was about 50% in men over 45 years within 8 years of developing angina and about half this in women. Patients with angina were also at higher risk of intermittent claudication, but the numbers were too small to assess the additional risk (if any) of stroke. Of the 57 men of the group just defined, 58% died during this period of follow-up, and of the 27 women 52%. Sudden death accounted for 44% of all these deaths. Overall in this study angina in men had a mortality of about 4% per year.

Resolution of anginal symptoms was also described in the Framingham study. There was a remission of new-onset angina pectoris for at least two years in 32% of men and 44% of women. Whether this represents a true resolution of symptoms or an original misdiagnosis is not known since the diagnosis was based on symptoms alone without cardiological investigation. In angina that had persisted before entry to the study for several years, the subsequent remission rates, 14% for men and 19% for women, were lower.

Israeli ischaemic heart disease study

In the Israeli ischaemic heart disease study, an occupational cohort of 9,764 healthy male civil service and municipal employees aged 40 years and over were followed up and diagnosed by physicians for definite or suspected angina pectoris, using a structured questionnaire.[5] The average annual incidence rate for angina pectoris alone was 5.7 per 1,000 or 7.2 per 1,000 (including those who presented with angina and evidence of clinical or 'silent' myocardial infarction), and incidence rose with age until 59 years and then plateaued. In contrast to the Framingham study, there were no intervening examinations between the baseline survey and 5-year follow-up, so this incidence rate may be an underestimate. Of the

256 men with definite new angina (without myocardial infarction) 85% were alive and well at five years, 7% suffered a myocardial infarction and 3% died from this cause, and the rest (5%) are unreported.[10] The risk of myocardial infarction for those with definite angina was twice that for those with no chest pain, and the relative risk of death for those with angina was fourfold.

Fry's general practice survey

John Fry's study of 260 patients with angina diagnosed and followed up in his London practice over 25 years is unique, not least because very few patients received treatment other than nitrates and no one had coronary artery surgery.[6] In most of these cases angina was the first presenting symptom of CHD; in a quarter, symptoms developed after a myocardial infarction. As in Framingham, there was a difference between the sexes, women having a much higher frequency of angina as a first symptom of CHD. Over the 25-year follow-up period, half the patients died, an annual mortality of 4.6%; the proportion of men and women who died was the same. Three quarters of these deaths were from cardiovascular causes. Of the survivors, 7% had had a myocardial infarction or developed congestive cardiac failure, 25% continued to have symptoms without complications, and in 18% there was complete resolution of symptoms. In those with persisting angina, it was only severe enough to cause pain on any exertion in one man; in 27% daily administration of glyceryl trinitrate was required and in the remaining 71% symptoms required only occasional or no glyceryl trinitrate tablets.

Edinburgh survey of new onset angina

A population survey of new and worsening angina was conducted in Edinburgh using a special clinic in the cardiology department at the Royal Infirmary over a period of $2\frac{1}{2}$ years.[7] Seventy-one selected general practitioners serving a population of 28,400 men (35–69 years) were asked to refer all men under 70 years of age who had experienced, during the preceding four weeks, chest pain suggestive of myocardial ischaemia that had occurred for the first time (new cases), had recurred after an interval of freedom of one month (recurrent), or had abruptly and unexpectedly increased in frequency or severity (exacerbation) in the absence of objective evidence of definite recent myocardial infarction. The criteria for new or worsening angina were met by 251 patients, of whom 21

had possible myocardial infarction with prolonged pain or equivocal ECG changes at their first visit. There were 129 patients who
had angina for the first time, of whom 10% had had a myocardial
infarction in the past. The incidence of serious cardiac complications (sudden death, definite or probable myocardial infarction or
resuscitated collapse) was 15.5% (39/251) for the whole population over 6 months. The rates of complications did not differ
between groups, being 14% (18/129) in those with new angina. Of
the 39 patients who suffered complications, 28 (72%) did so within
6 months and 34 (87%) within 12 weeks of the onset of symptoms.
Of these serious cardiac complications, 9 (4%) were deaths and 30
(12%) developed myocardial infarction but survived. Of those who
survived without myocardial infarction, 66 (31%) had no angina at
6 months.

The clinical selection of patients for in-hospital investigation and
treatment was no better than the play of chance in relation to
prognosis. Eighty-seven patients were admitted to hospital because
of prolonged chest pain or progressive worsening of angina, of
whom 18.4% (10) had serious cardiac complications up to 6
months after their initial referral to a special clinic. This complica-
tion rate did not differ significantly from that of the 23 (14%) who
were not admitted to hospital but had serious cardiac complications over the same period.

A discriminant function analysis (including age, pattern of pain,
history of myocardial infarction, ECG ST segment or T wave
changes, cardiothoracic ratio, blood pressure and other risk factors
for CHD) could only predict one third of these cases with an
unfavourable prognosis. As in the Framingham study, the Edinburgh survey was based on a clinical history and resting ECG only,
as exercise tests were performed only where the diagnosis was in
doubt. Coronary arteriography was not undertaken in any case.

Southampton chest pain clinic survey

Our survey in Southampton was based on a chest pain clinic which
offered an open access service to a random sample of 17 practices
(117 general practitioners) serving an adult population of 192,000
men and women.[8] General practitioners agreed to refer *all* new
patients less than 70 years of age to our clinic who presented for
the first time with chest pain that in the opinion of the general
practitioner could be due to CHD. Patients with a history of CHD
were excluded and those with suspected unstable angina or
myocardial infarction were admitted directly to hospital by the

general practitioner in the usual way. More than 95% of patients referred to the clinic were assessed by a cardiology registrar within 24 hours of seeing their general practitioner.

A full history was taken followed by a clinical examination, blood sample, resting ECG, exercise tolerance test and a chest X-ray. The patient was classified as having definite angina on the basis of the following criteria: (i) recurrent, (ii) brief (up to 15 minutes) episodes of chest pain, (iii) precipitated by exertion or exertion and emotion, (iv) relieved by rest or glyceryl trinitrate and (v) the character and radiation of which were consistent with the diagnosis. When some, but not all characteristics were present, the patient was classified as 'possible angina'. The duration of symptoms in definite angina cases varied: 39% reported symptoms for less than a month, 36% for 1–4 months, 15% for 4–12 months, and in 10% symptoms had been present for more than a year. Angina was experienced daily by 34%, symptoms occurred at least once a week in 52% and less frequently than this in the remainder.

A total of 467 patients were referred between October 1990 and March 1992, of whom 62% were male (median age 52) and 38% were female (median age 55). Of the total, 110 (24%) had definite angina (63% male, 33% female) and 63 (13%) possible angina (62% male, 38% female); their classification is shown in Fig. 1. Patients with *definite* or *possible* angina had 1 mm horizontal/downsloping ST depression on their resting electrocardiogram in 5% and in none respectively; Q/QS patterns in 4% and in none; complete left bundle branch block in one patient with definite and one with possible angina, and right bundle branch block in one with definite and two with possible angina. In patients with definite or possible angina who underwent exercise electrocardiography ischaemia (≥ 1 mm ST depression) was provoked in 61% and 32% respectively. In the definite angina group, 29% (30/103) had marked ischaemia (≥ 3 mm horizontal/downsloping ST depression) on exercise testing. The duration of symptoms, age, gender, body mass index, smoking habit, diastolic blood pressure and blood cholesterol were not related in logistic regression analysis to severity of ischaemia on exercise.

A handwritten preliminary report summarising the clinical findings, investigations and recommended management was given to the patient for delivery to the general practitioner. The recommendations for management covered modification of risk factors, medical therapy and, where appropriate on the basis of exercise test result, referral to the regional cardiac centre for coronary arteriography. With a few exceptions the ultimate responsibility for referral

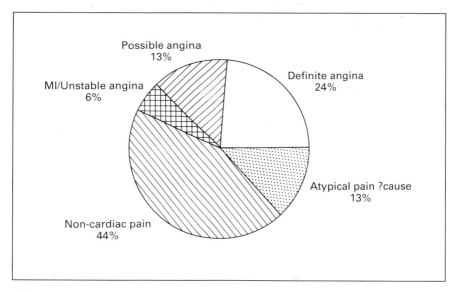

Fig. 1. *Clinical classification of referrals; n=467.*

was left to the patient's general practitioner who thus retained control over the patient's management and choice of consultant. A full typewritten summary was posted to the general practitioner within 7 days of referral in 72% of cases and in 90% within 2 weeks.

The referral rate to the chest pain clinic was 193 patients per 100,000 patient population under 70 years of age per year. The age- and sex-specific incidence rates for definite angina, given in Table 2, show a rise in incidence with age in both men and women, the frequency being higher in men, although not in middle age, with twice as many cases in the oldest age group of 61–70 years. The incidence in men aged 61–70 years was five times higher than that in those aged 31–40. When these rates are applied to the

Table 2. Age and sex incidence rates per 1,000 per annum (95% confidence intervals).

	Age (years)				
	31–40	41–50	51–60	61–70	Total
Men	0.44	0.43	1.32	2.32	1.13
	(0.09, 0.80)	(0.05, 0.31)	(0.57, 2.07)	(1.27, 3.36)	(0.85, 1.40)
Women	0.08	0.56	1.05	1.01	0.53
	(0, 0.25)	(0.1, 1.01)	(0.36, 1.73)	(0.35, 1.67)	(0.33, 0.72)

UK population, with the assumption that the same disease frequency will be experienced throughout the country, a total of 22,570 (15,250 men and 7,320 women) new definite angina cases (<70 years of age) might be expected annually; about 13,980 (9,730 men and 4,250 women) will have ischaemia (≥1 mm ST depression) on exercise testing, and 6,790 (4,690 men and 2,100 women) will have sufficiently severe evidence of ischaemia (≥3 mm ST depression) to justify coronary arteriography.

Conclusion

In measuring frequency and prognosis, surveys of angina should be undertaken in the general population, to avoid the inherent biases in selected hospital patients. Study of incident cases and their clinical course and prognosis will give the complete clinical picture.

Only five population surveys have reported incidence rates for angina, and four of them were published nearly two decades ago. In these studies the crude incidence rates of new angina in men, which ranged from 0.59 to 5.7 (a ninefold difference), may reflect real variation in CHD experience between these populations, but differences in their age/gender structure, diagnostic criteria for angina (and whether or not other manifestations of CHD were included), temporal changes in incidence, and statistical confidence in estimating rates must also be taken into account. In our Southampton survey the incidence of new definite angina rose with age, and in men and women the crude rates (95% CI) were 1.13 (0.85, 1.40) and 0.53 (0.33, 0.72) per 1,000 per annum respectively. Application of the age-specific rates to the UK population as a whole would yield 22,570 new cases of angina per annum in men and women under 70 years of age. About two thirds of new cases will have objective evidence of ischaemia (≥1 mm ST depression) on exercise testing, and just under one third will have ischaemia of sufficient severity (≥3 mm ST depression) to justify coronary arteriography.

It is not easy to summarise prognosis of angina from these population surveys since there is a range of serious cardiac complications, in rate and scale, which may be real or due to differences in methods. What is clear is that survival for men (and possibly women) with angina is poorer than for the general healthy population, and that there is no reliable way of predicting those who go on to develop unstable angina or myocardial infarction or die. In a significant minority of patients, symptoms are reported to resolve, but this apparently benign prognosis needs to be verified in patients with coronary artery disease confirmed angiographically, since a likely explanation for this course of events is misdiagnosis.

Management of angina in our population is still largely the responsibility of general practitioners, with only a small minority of patients referred for a specialist opinion.[11] Treatment is usually medical; cardiological tests beyond a resting ECG are uncommon. Although coronary arteriography is the only investigation that can identify the patients most likely to benefit from surgical revascularisation, it is undertaken in very few patients at the time of presentation. The clinical challenge is to identify cases of angina in the population, describe their clinical characteristics using modern cardiological investigations, and then develop measures to predict more confidently progression to unstable angina, myocardial infarction and sudden death. Medical and surgical treatments could then be tested in randomised trials to determine whether, in such patients predicted to be a high risk, the morbidity and mortality of this common disease can be reduced.

References

1. Rose GA. Ischaemic heart disease: chest pain questionnaire. *Milbank Memorial Fund Quarterly* 1965; **43**: 32–9.
2. Shaper AG, Cook DG, Walker M, MacFarlane PW. Prevalence of ischaemic heart disease in middle aged British men. *British Heart Journal* 1984; **51**: 595–606.
3. Rose G, Baxter PJ, Reid DD, McCartney P. Prevalence and prognosis of electrocardiographic findings in middle-aged men. *British Heart Journal* 1978; **40**: 636–43.
4. Kannel WB, Feinleib M. Natural history of angina pectoris in the Framingham study: prognosis and survival. *American Journal of Cardiology* 1972; **29**: 154–63.
5. Medalie JH, Snyder M, Groen JJ, Neufeld HN, Goldbourt U, Riss E. Angina pectoris among 10,000 men: 5 year incidence and univariate analysis. *American Journal of Medicine* 1973; **55**: 583–94.
6. Fry J. The natural history of angina in a general practice. *Journal of the Royal College of General Practitioners* 1976; **26**: 643–6.
7. Duncan B, Fulton M, Morrison SL, Lutz W, Donald KW, Kerr F, Kirby BJ, Julian DG, Oliver MF. Prognosis of new and worsening angina pectoris. *British Medical Journal* 1976; **1**: 981–5.
8. Gandhi MM, Lampe F, Wood DA. Incidence of stable angina pectoris. *European Heart Journal* 1992; **13**: 181.
9. Kannell WB, Sorlie PD. Remission of clinical angina pectoris: the Framingham study. *American Journal of Cardiology* 1978; **42**: 119–23.
10. Medalie JH, Goldbourt U. Angina pectoris among 10,000 men. II. Psychosocial and other risk factors as evidenced by a multivariate analysis of a five year incidence study. *American Journal of Medicine* 1976; **60**: 910–21.

11. Cannon PJ, Cannell PA, Stockley IH, Garner ST, Hampton JR. Preva-
    lence of angina as assessed by a survey of prescriptions for nitrates.
    Lancet 1988; **1**: 979–81.

3 | Prevalence of angina in the community

John Hampton
Professor of Cardiology, University Hospital, Nottingham

Coronary artery disease can be asymptomatic, or may manifest itself as sudden death, myocardial infarction, or angina. Asymptomatic disease is obviously important but it is almost impossible to study its prevalence. There is a natural tendency to assume that studying one of the clinical syndromes associated with coronary atheroma will provide information relevant to the others, but this is not necessarily so. Although atheroma underlies all the coronary syndromes, the major events—sudden death and myocardial infarction—are probably more related to thrombosis, while angina may result from progressive arterial narrowing which does not necessarily have a thrombotic component. It would be highly convenient to assume that the coronary syndromes would all be closely associated in time and space, but such evidence as exists suggests that this may not be so.[1] Most epidemiological studies have been concerned with major events because they are easy to identify, and it is difficult to be sure how much of the temporal and geographical discrepancy between them and angina relates to different degrees of difficulty in identifying these three syndromes (angina, myocardial infarction and sudden death) in large population groups.

National and international patterns of death from coronary diseases have been studied in great detail on the basis of death certificates which, although of doubtful accuracy in individual cases, probably give a reasonable indication of the cause of death in large populations. The changing mortality trends in the Western world have been well documented, if not well explained. Mortality from coronary disease began to fall in the USA in the early 1960s,[2] and rather later in the UK. Although changes in the International Classification of Diseases (ICD) codes in their 7th and 8th revisions resulted in changes in the absolute numbers of deaths classified as due to coronary disease, these discontinuities can be seen to be unimportant as year by year data have accumulated, and there can be little doubt that the decline in mortality is real. Equally, there can be little doubt that within the UK there is marked regional variation in major coronary events, with the North and West being much more severely affected than the South and East.[3] The relationship of risk factors such as smoking, blood cholesterol level and blood pressure to major risk events has been studied in great detail, with similar findings, in the USA, the UK, Israel and elsewhere.[4-7] It has been shown in the USA that the change in death rate cannot easily be explained by changes in the conventional risk factors,[8] so the precise importance of risk factors remains unclear.

Unfortunately there is no equivalent of the death certificate for angina, and because the diagnosis of angina is not easy we cannot make any confident statements about its prevalence in one country as compared with another, about changes in its incidence and prevalence over the past two decades, or about the relative importance of different risk factors.

Purpose of angina surveys

There are several reasons why it would be helpful to know as much about angina as we do about major coronary events. The main purpose of epidemiology is to generate testable hypotheses about mechanisms of disease, so if we know precisely how the prevalence of angina relates to that of major coronary events we might have some indication whether similar or different disease mechanisms are involved. If we could relate geographical differences or temporal changes in angina prevalence to differences in risk factors, it might be possible to disentangle causal relationships and mere association. At a more pragmatic level, prevalence studies of angina would help the planning of services, and would highlight deficiencies in different parts of the country. It has been shown that the prevalence of angina is the main risk factor for a subsequent event,[5,9] so prevalence studies might give an early warning of the need for services such as percutaneous transluminal coronary angiography (PTCA) and coronary artery bypass grafting (CABG). Whether or not early detection and treatment have contributed to the decline in mortality from heart disease is a matter of debate,[10] but if there were any treatment that undoubtedly reduced fatality in patients with angina, it would be important to identify individual patients in the community as well as to obtain an overall picture of the incidence and prevalence of the problem.

Unfortunately the diagnosis of angina is not easy. It is one of the main problems that cardiologists have to deal with daily; even with sophisticated and expensive aids like treadmill testing (Chapter 5), thallium scintigraphy (Chapter 9), and coronary angiography

(Chapter 6), a definite diagnosis can be difficult to achieve. Community surveys have to make do with far more simple measures, and epidemiologists tend to be satisfied with techniques sufficiently standardised to allow populations to be compared, without worrying too much about the precision of their diagnosis.

Techniques for angina surveys

Epidemiological methods that are to be applied to large populations have to be simple and cheap, and the techniques mainly used are a description of a patient's previous history, a questionnaire about current symptoms, and some form of resting electrocardiogram (ECG). All of these have limitations, and none is as simple or quick as identifying ischaemic heart disease death certificates. Because of these difficulties, most surveys have been limited to specific age groups, or to 'captive' populations in particular employments.

Asking patients to recall previous diagnoses gives results that appear unreliable. In the survey of men from 24 British towns (see below) the subjects were asked if they had ever been told that they had heart disease.[11] Of 7,727 men, 424 (5.5%) recalled that a doctor had once told them that they had angina or a heart attack. However, only one third of those who, on direct questioning, gave a history suggestive that a heart attack had occurred remembered such a diagnosis being made. Only half of those with a definite myocardial infarction on their ECG could remember a diagnosis suggesting coronary disease. Even among those with apparently severe angina, only 40% had been diagnosed by a doctor. Presumably in many cases the men had never consulted a doctor, so there had been no chance for a diagnostic label to be attached, but men who have chest pain at the time of one survey have frequently lost it when questioned again after a few years, and may deny that they ever have pain. Rose interviewed 1,136 men in 1961 and interviewed 995 of them again in 1962.[12] The prevalence rates for angina were 3.3% and 3.4% in 1961 and 1962 respectively, but the men who made up the groups were different. Approximately half of those with angina in 1961 (19 of 33) did not have it in 1962, and nearly half (14 of 32) of those whose answers were positive in 1962 had given negative answers in 1961. Therefore neither asking a patient about previous symptoms or diagnoses, nor surveying general practitioner records, is likely to give an accurate estimate of angina prevalence.

Estimating incidence is even more difficult: although the Israeli

ischaemic heart disease study[13] estimated an incidence rate in middle-aged men of 5.7 per 1,000, this was based on a 5-year period
when presumably quite a lot of those surveyed would have developed angina, lost it, and forgotten they ever had it (see Chapter 2).

Questionnaires designed to identify patients with angina, such as
that designed by Rose, have been used in a number of studies.[14,15]
Unfortunately questionnaires lack specificity and sensitivity in making a diagnosis, even if their results are reproducible. Use of the
Rose questionnaire indicates a higher prevalence of angina in
women than in men, but it is not clear whether this is true,
whether women have an increased sensitivity to pain, or whether
they simply describe symptoms that are really due to anxiety.[16]

The ECG is not an easy survey tool because of the time each
recording takes, and the difficulty of standardising its interpretation. Strict use of a diagnostic system such as the Minnesota code
increases reproducibility, but reproducibility of diagnosis perhaps
becomes of secondary importance when the need to record many
ECGs leads to the use of simple systems such as limb leads only[9] or
an orthogonal lead,[5] since neither of these would be acceptable to
a cardiologist dealing with an individual patient. Worse, the ECG is
not a constant phenomenon even within an individual patient, for
T-wave abnormalities can be evanescent, and even Q-waves due to
myocardial infarction can disappear with the passage of time.

All these difficulties being accepted, such techniques have been
used effectively in surveys for angina, and it is worth considering
the major studies that have been performed in the United
Kingdom.

British angina surveys

The Whitehall study of cardiac disease involved 18,403 male civil
servants aged 40–64 working in or near Whitehall.[14,17] The study
can therefore immediately be seen to have had limitations: it
applied to middle-aged males only, and those living in the South
East of England where the standardised mortality ratio for
ischaemic heart disease is relatively low. The men were investigated
between 1967 and 1969 by means of a self-administered questionnaire and a limb lead ECG; 3,770 (20.5%) had some evidence of
ischaemic heart disease (1,143 with an ischaemic ECG, 1,908 with a
positive questionnaire, and 719 already being under medical care).

The World Health Organisation multifactorial trial in the prevention of coronary heart disease included a UK group (the UK
Heart Disease Prevention Project) which surveyed 18,210 men

aged 40–59 years employed in 24 factories between 1971 and 1973.[18] Positive answers were given by 10.2% to a questionnaire about symptoms of ischaemic heart disease, and 7.8% had an abnormal ECG.

The British regional heart survey[5] studied the prevalence of ischaemic heart disease by questionnaire and ECG in 7,735 men aged 40–59 years selected at random from general practices in 24 British towns. One quarter of the men had some evidence of ischaemic heart disease; on questionnaire alone, 14% had angina or had had a possible myocardial infarction, and 15% had an abnormal ECG with 4% showing a previous infarction. Half of those with a possible infarction or angina on questionnaire had a normal ECG and half of those with ECG evidence of a previous infarction had never had chest pain. Table 1 summarises the results of these studies.

Table 1. Prevalence of ischaemic heart disease (IHD) in the Whitehall study, the UK heart disease prevention project (UKHDPP) and the British regional heart study (RHS).

Diagnostic category	Whitehall (1967–9) Civil Service men 40–64	UKHDPP (1971–3) Factories men 40–59	RHS (1978–80) Random men 40–59
By questionnaire			
Angina	4.3	3.6	7.9
Possible MI	6.5	6.6	9.1
Either	10.4	–	14.2
By ECG			
Major ischaemia	0.5	0.9	3.1
Other	5.0	6.9	11.4
Any evidence of IHD	14.1	–	24.7

The British regional study produced the highest figures for angina prevalence in the UK; this may have been due to differences in the ECG technique, or may have resulted from all those in the Whitehall study still being at work with the sick ones having retired. Other important differences may have been social class, and the different geographical areas studied.

Surveys of patients under treatment for ischaemic heart disease

In the Whitehall study, which it must be remembered was only of middle-aged employed men, 719 patients (3.8% of those surveyed) were under medical care but more than 96% were not. Surveys limited to patients being treated for ischaemic heart disease clearly have a different purpose from population studies. They start with the assumption that the important patients are those whose symptoms have been severe enough for them to seek help from a doctor, and this assumption is probably not unreasonable. In the Whitehall study,[9] the patients already under medical care had a 5-year fatality of 8.9%, but for those whose only positive finding was an ischaemic ECG or a positive questionnaire the 5-year fatality rates were 3.3% and 2.5% respectively. Studies of patients under care therefore have the virtue of being the simplest way of predicting future major events.

The main use of these studies, however, is to obtain data for the planning of services rather than to obtain epidemiological data that may illuminate mechanisms of disease. In theory, the identification of patients is easy since they are recorded in hospital or general practitioner records. Where computerised diagnostic registers are maintained, finding these patients should indeed be simple, but unless registers are maintained for research purposes it is unlikely that they will be either complete or accurate.

Heart attack registers have been maintained for relatively brief periods in Oxford,[19] Edinburgh,[20] Tower Hamlets,[21] and for nearly 20 years in Nottingham.[22] They have mainly been hospital-based, though in Nottingham an attempt was made to identify patients with suspected heart attacks who were cared for at home. The sudden nature of heart attack symptoms, and the dramatic events that follow, make such registers much easier to obtain than a register of patients with angina.

Patients referred to hospital with chronic chest pain clearly form such a selected group that, even in areas with apparently high referral rates,[23] hospital data tell us little about angina in the community. In an attempt to predict the likely demand for coronary surgery, the Royal College of General Practitioners established a survey of patients being treated for angina by 51 general practitioners in Newcastle; this involved a population of 125,000 patients, and the survey was made over a 4-month period in 1979.[24] The general practitioners recorded all the patients they treated who were aged 30–59, and concluded that the prevalence of angina in their population was 1.1%.

The Nottingham nitrate survey

Most patients with angina are likely to be treated with a nitrate. Nitrates are seldom used for the treatment of any disease other than angina, and short-acting nitrates need to be replaced frequently. We made the hypothesis that, if all prescriptions for nitrates issued within the Nottingham district health authority in a 6-month period could be obtained, we would be able to establish the number of patients with angina sufficiently severe to need medical treatment, and thereby establish the number of patients known to general practitioners who might need to be referred to hospital for detailed investigation and specialist treatment.

The most commonly prescribed nitrate preparations were identified from national sales figures. Copies of prescriptions for these and for a dermal nitrate preparation that were issued by general practitioners in the Nottingham health district from October 1984 to March 1985 (inclusive) were obtained from the Prescription Pricing Authority (PPA). The prescriptions for nitrates issued in the outpatient departments of Nottingham hospitals during this period were obtained from the pharmacy files.

The patients' names and addresses were recorded on a microcomputer with software that allowed identification of repeat prescriptions for individual patients.

Men older than 65 years and women older than 60 years receive free medication in the UK, and if the patient's age is above these limits it is indicated on the prescription form (FP10). This information, details of other drugs prescribed simultaneously and the name of the general practitioner or hospital doctor were also recorded on the database.

The PPA identified 15,242 prescriptions for nitrates issued by general practitioners, and hospital pharmacy files showed that 509 had been issued by the Nottingham hospitals. There were 300 illegible prescriptions which had to be discarded. The 15,451 prescriptions remaining related to 6,856 patients, of whom 6,421 received prescriptions only from general practitioners; 435 patients received prescriptions from hospitals, and of those 231 also received prescriptions from general practitioners (Table 2).

A nitrate alone was prescribed for 4,326 patients (63%) (2,799 being given only a short-acting preparation), although it is possible that other drugs were prescribed separately; 377 patients (5.7%) (Table 3) received prescriptions for nitrates, beta-blockers and calcium antagonists simultaneously, and 254 of these (4% of the whole group) were treated with a long-acting nitrate. These

254 patients are presumably the ones with the most severe angina.

Specificity

To establish the specificity of nitrate prescription analysis for angina (ie the percentage of patients identified who actually had angina) a random 10% sample of the general practitioners in the Nottingham health district was taken and an attempt was made to review their records of all the patients for whom they prescribed nitrates. These records were scrutinised for evidence of angina, and for information about investigations and referral to hospital clinics. A patient was judged to have definite angina if there was a

Table 2. Nottingham nitrate survey; age and sex distribution of patients identified from nitrate prescriptions.

	Identification source			
Age group	GP only	Hospital only	Hospital and GP	Total patients
Male <65	1,351	81	82	1,514
Male ≥65	1,755	33	50	1,838
Female <60	438	18	24	480
Female ≥60	2,259	45	70	2,374
Age/sex not known	618	27	5	650
Total	*6,421*	*204*	*231*	*6,856*

Table 3. Nottingham nitrate survey; number of patients prescribed other anti-anginal agents in addition to nitrates.

Age group	Beta-blocker	Calcium antagonist	Beta-blocker and calcium antagonist
Male <65	462 (31%)	138 (9%)	191 (13%)
Male ≥65	442 (24%)	113 (6%)	64 (3%)
Female <60	101 (21%)	34 (7%)	34 (7%)
Female ≥60	555 (23%)	134 (6%)	69 (3%)
Age not stated	142 (22%)	32 (5%)	19 (3%)
Total	*1,702*	*451*	*377*

record of a convincing story plus a record of an abnormal coronary arteriogram, an abnormal exercise test, or an ischaemic ECG
recorded during a period of pain. In the case of hospital patients
who died, definite angina was considered to have been present if
they satisfied these criteria, or if necropsy showed coronary disease. Patients were considered to have probable angina if they gave
a convincing history and had either an ischaemic ECG at rest, or
an ECG showing left bundle branch block. Patients were recorded
as having possible angina if the diagnosis depended purely on the
patient's history, without supporting evidence.

During the survey period, 636 patients received prescriptions for
nitrates from the 28 general practitioners randomly selected for the
assessment of specificity of the survey technique. The records of 137
patients could not be found, so 499 were inspected. In all but 21,
the general practitioner considered the patient to have angina. Of
the remaining 478 patients for whom records could be retrieved, 29
(6%) were considered to have definite angina, 162 (32%) probable
angina, and 287 (57%) possible angina. Analysis of nitrate prescriptions is thus 96% specific for a diagnosis of angina.

Sensitivity

To establish the sensitivity of the nitrate prescription survey for the
prevalence of patients with treated angina, ie the percentage of
patients under treatment who were identified by the survey, the
records of two practices with computerised repeat prescription systems, and three with diagnostic registers, were examined. The
patients identified in this way were compared with those from the
same practice who were identified by the nitrate prescription survey.

The five practices with either a computerised prescription system or a diagnostic index were large practices and together served
a population of 37,753 patients. A considerable variation of sensitivity was detected, from 46% to 92%, with a mean of 73%. This
probably related to differences in the way in which patients with
angina were recorded in each practice rather than to variations in
angina prevalence between practices.

Overall, the prescription survey identified 307 (73%) of the 420
patients considered by their general practitioners to have angina,
so the average sensitivity of this technique was 73%.

Prevalence of angina

The total of 6,856 patients in the Nottingham health district identified from the nitrate prescription survey is presumably a slight overestimate of the prevalence of angina because the specificity of the survey is 96%; on the other hand, it could be a considerable underestimate because the sensitivity may be as low as 73%. If we accept these estimates of specificity and sensitivity, the prevalence of angina in the Nottingham health district is approximately 9,000 in a population of 612,800, or 1.5%. Because a prescription reveals a patient's age group, not the precise age, only limited information can be obtained about angina prevalence and age. In the Nottingham health district there are 344,700 people aged over 30 years; if we assume that no patient under this age has angina, the prevalence in individuals aged over 30 years is 2.6%. Table 4 shows the calculated prevalence of angina for men below and above age 65, and for women below and above age 60, excluding individuals under the age of 30.

Table 4. Nottingham nitrate survey; estimated number of patients in different age groups with treated angina in Nottingham district health authority.

Age group	Number of patients in nitrate survey	Estimated number of patients with treated angina	Age-corrected prevalence
Male <65	1,514	1,991	1.5%
Male ≥65	1,838	2,417	7.1%
Female <60	480	631	0.6%
Female ≥60	2,374	3,122	4.4%
Age not stated	650	855	–
Total	6,856	9,016	–

Total population in Nottingham district health authority 612,800.

Use of investigations and hospital services

Most the of 499 patients for whom the 10% sample of general practitioners prescribed nitrates had not been investigated in detail. Only 320 (64%) had had an ECG, 34 (7%) had had an exercise test, and 19 (4%) had had a coronary angiogram. Of these 499 patients, 96 (19%) attended a hospital medical clinic during the 6-month study period, and half of these were seen by a cardiologist.

A separate search of the hospital main index computer file showed that 1,770 (26%) of the total survey population had been seen by a medical or geriatric consultant as either an inpatient or an outpatient between 1 January 1981 and 31 March 1985.

Conclusion

Angina is common, variable over time, and difficult to diagnose with simple questionnaires and tests. Establishing the incidence and prevalence of angina in a community is clearly of academic interest; if we could be sure that any intervention prolonged life it would be of considerable clinical importance. Surveys aimed at limited populations (the employed, those under 65 years and so on) will inevitably underestimate the size of the problem. The prevalence of angina is likely to increase with the ageing population, and perhaps particularly in some subgroups such as ageing Asian men. Increased public awareness and an increased use of health screening can be expected to lead to an increase in hospital workload.

For all these reasons it is difficult to identify precisely what level of investigational and specialised treatment facilities will be needed. It is, however, quite clear that already many patients with clinically significant angina (as opposed to chest pain discovered only on screening) are being treated in the community without referral to hospital for detailed assessment.

References

1. Smith WCS, Kenicer MB, Tunstall-Pedoe H, Clark EC, Crombie IK. Prevalence of coronary heart disease in Scotland: Scottish Heart Health Study. *British Heart Journal* 1990; **64**: 295–8.
2. Ragland KA, Selvin S, Merrill DW. The onset of decline in ischemic heart disease mortality in the United States. *American Journal of Epidemiology* 1988; **127**: 516–31.
3. Elford J, Phillips AN, Thomson AG, Shaper AG. Migration and geographic variations in ischaemic heart disease in Great Britain. *Lancet* 1989; **i**: 343–6.
4. Dawber TR. *The Framingham Study: the epidemiology of atherosclerotic disease.* Cambridge, Mass.: Harvard University Press, 1980.
5. Shaper AG, Cook DG, Walker M, Macfarlane PW. Prevalence of ischaemic heart disease in middle aged British men. *British Heart Journal* 1984; **51**: 595–605.
6. Ragland DR, Brand RJ. Coronary heart disease mortality in the Western Collaborative Group Study. *American Journal of Epidemiology* 1988; **127**: 462–75.
7. Medalie JH, Kahn HA, Neufeld HN *et al.* Myocardial infarction among 10,000 adult males over a 5 year period. I. Prevalence incidence and mortality experience. *Journal of Chronic Disease* 1973; **26**: 63.

8. Kaplan GA, Cohn BA, Cohen RD, Guralnik J. The decline in ischemic heart disease mortality: prospective evidence from the Alameda County Study. *American Journal of Epidemiology* 1988; **127**: 1131–42.

9. Rose G, Baxter PJ, Reid DD, McCartney P. Prevalence and prognosis of electrocardiographic findings in middle-aged men. *British Heart Journal* 1978; **40**: 636–43.

10. Cohn BA, Kaplan GA, Cohen RD. Did early detection and treatment contribute to the decline in ischemic heart disease mortality? Prospective evidence from the Alameda County Study. *American Journal of Epidemiology* 1988; **127**: 1143–54.

11. Shaper AG, Cook DG, Walker M, Macfarlane PW. Recall of diagnosis by men with ischaemic heart disease. *British Heart Journal* 1984; **51**: 606–11.

12. Rose GA. Ischaemic heart disease. Chest pain questionnaire. *Milbank Memorial Fund Quarterly* 1965; **43**: 32–9.

13. Medalie JA, Goldbourt U. Angina pectoris among 10,000 men. II. Psychosocial and other risk factors as evidenced by a multivariate analysis of a five year incidence study. *American Journal of Medicine* 1976; **60**: 910–21.

14. Reid DD, Brett GZ, Hamilton PJS, Jarrett RJ, Keen H, Rose G. Cardiorespiratory disease and diabetes among middle-aged male civil servants: a study of screening and intervention. *Lancet* 1974; **i**: 469–73.

15. Abernathy JR, Thorn MD, Trobaugh GB *et al.* Prevalence of ischemic resting and stress electrocardiographic abnormalities and angina among 40–59-year-old men in selected US and USSR populations. *Circulation* 1988; **77**: 270–8.

16. Wilcosky T, Harris R, Weissfeld L. The prevalence and correlates of Rose questionnaire angina among women and men in the lipid research clinics program prevalence study population. *American Journal of Epidemiology* 1987; **125**: 400–9.

17. Rose G, Reid DD, Hamilton PJS, McCartney P, Keen H, Jarrett RJ. Myocardial ischaemia, risk factors and death from coronary heart disease. *Lancet* 1977; **i**: 105–9.

18. WHO European Collaborative Group. Multifactorial trial in the prevention of coronary heart disease. I. Recruitment and critical findings. *European Heart Journal* 1980; **1**: 73–80.

19. Kinlen LJ. Incidence and presentation of myocardial infarction in an English community. *British Heart Journal* 1973; **35**: 616–22.

20. Armstrong A, Duncan B, Oliver MF *et al.* Natural history of acute coronary heart attacks: a community study. *British Heart Journal* 1972; **34**: 67–80.

21. Pedoe HT, Clayton D, Morris JN, Brigden W, McDonald L. Coronary heart attacks in East London. *Lancet* 1975; **ii**: 833–8.

22. Rowley JM, Mounser P, Harrison EA, Skene AM, Hampton JR. The management of myocardial infarction: implications for current policy derived from the Nottingham heart attack register. *British Heart Journal* 1991; **67**: 255–62.

23. Cripps T, Dennis MS, Joy M. The need for invasive cardiological assessment and operation: viewpoint of a district general hospital. *British Heart Journal* 1986; **55**: 488–93.

24. Research Committee, Northern General Faculty, Royal College of General Practitioners. Study of angina in patients aged 30–59 in general practice. *British Medical Journal* 1982; **285**: 1319–21.

4 | What a general practitioner wants from a referral service for suspected angina

John K Inman
General Practitioner, The Health Centre,
Melton Road, Syston, Leicester

Most patients who attend hospital for any specialty do so having been referred by their general practitioner. Indeed, the important role of the general practitioner as gatekeeper and proxy for the patient is acknowledged in the National Health Service and Community Care Act 1990. In this chapter I consider the scale and diversity of problems faced in general practice when managing patients with suspected angina.

Background

A survey by the Royal College of General Practitioners published in 1986 demonstrated the incidence rates of different manifestations

Table 1. Incidence of coronary heart disease; males and females by age; England and Wales 1981/82; rates per 1,000 population.[1]

Age	Men			Women		
	Acute myocardial infarction	Angina of effort	Other coronary heart disease	Acute myocardial infarction	Angina of effort	Other coronary heart disease
15–24	0.0	–	0.1	–	–	–
25–44	0.8	0.3	0.2	0.2	0.4	0.1
45–64	7.4	6.8	3.6	2.5	4.4	1.6
65–74	12.8	14.2	6.9	6.8	9.0	5.5
>75	13.9	14.4	8.4	9.2	9.5	6.8
All ages	*3.4*	*3.3*	*1.8*	*1.9*	*2.6*	*1.4*

of coronary heart disease.[1] Further data from this report suggest that 1.6% of the population of England and Wales (ie 814,000 people) consult their family doctor during the course of the year because of coronary heart disease.

Population data from the Office of Population Censuses and Surveys (1985) combined with data from the Royal College of General Practitioners predict a total of 34,000 new cases of coronary heart disease in general practice per annum in England and Wales.[2] Of this total, about 27% of new events involve males aged 45–64 years, who themselves account for only 11% of the population as a whole.

John Fry, a general practitioner, recorded 776 new cases of coronary heart disease (including angina, myocardial infarction and sudden death) in his practice over the 35 years from 1947. The annual population incidence worked out at six per thousand per year (male:female ratio 2.5:1).[3] Of all the new cases of coronary heart disease presenting in his practice in that period, 28% had angina, 55% had a myocardial infarct and 17% suffered sudden death. From these data, general practitioners with an average list size of 2,500 might expect 10–15 new cases of coronary heart disease to present each year. In addition each may have 50–75 persons with a past history of coronary heart disease, of whom 25–30 will consult him or her in any one year.

Another general practitioner, Keith Hodgkin, kept detailed records of all his patient contacts from his time as a medical student throughout his professional career.[4] He recorded an incidence of coronary heart disease of 6.7–8.5 per 1,000 National Health Service patients per year (male/female ratio 2:1). The epidemiology is further considered in Chapters 2 and 3, and by Tunstall-Pedoe.[5]

Absolute figures of incidence and attack rates are impossible to obtain, for in every community there must be unreported morbidity never seen by any doctor.

Problems with presentation

Coronary heart disease clearly constitutes a substantial part of the workload of general practitioners, either through genuine disease or effects on the 'worried well'.

There are many causes of chest pain in a patient presenting in general practice, but many sufferers fear coronary disease to be the cause. The media encourage people (perhaps correctly) to equate chest pain with heart disease. Fortunately, the experienced practitioner can often immediately and properly reassure the patient as to a non-cardiac cause after taking a simple history and subsequent examination. However, it is important to realise that asymptomatic coronary arterial atheromatous disease as an occult disease process can never be excluded. In one study of presentation of chest pain in general practice nearly half the cases were attributed to the musculoskeletal system.[6] In some cases examination may reveal an obvious cause such as the rash of shingles.

The real problem arises when a patient presents with thoracic sensations that are not typical of angina. In this situation anxiety and uncertainty may be fostered in both patient and physician. This is further compounded by the fact that the usual diagnostic procedures such as physical examination, chest X-ray and resting ECG may be normal in the presence of coronary artery disease and thus cannot be relied upon to resolve the problem of differential diagnosis. So to what extent can a correct diagnosis be deduced from the history?

The history

Many researchers have studied the predictive accuracy of pointers from the history. Master in 1964 reported on 200 consecutively studied patients with chest pain in whom he suspected significant coronary artery disease and 200 patients similarly judged to be free of coronary disease.[7] He studied the distribution of age, the site, quality and duration of the pain, its radiation, time scale, precipitating factors, frequency of episodes and the response to glyceryl trinitrate. He concluded that the distinction between cardiac and non-cardiac chest pain is often not possible by history alone. However, although he felt that no single feature could be considered as characteristic of coronary disease or non-coronary disease, not surprisingly he stated that the chances of distinction are increased when there are multiple characteristic factors. Hodgkin looked at patients with anginal symptoms (characteristic chest pains) and found that 50% of these experienced classical radiation to the arms or jaw, 80% noted pain on exertion and 65% complained of dyspnoea.[8]

Standardised questionnaires have some advantages for studying the epidemiology of angina by reducing observer variability, and they are easy to administer.[9,10] However, their validation is indirect and incomplete because the number of false positives and false negatives cannot be known. Even when an ECG is abnormal this does not disprove a negative assessment from the questionnaire. The method is further confounded by the apparently spontaneous recovery from, and development of, angina in some patients. In one study by Fry in general practice, follow-up of 200 persons diagnosed as having angina showed that 24% ceased to suffer pain altogether over 25 years of observation.[3]

Another study found that patients with 'definite' or 'possible' angina, as determined by questionnaire, had a much higher prevalence rate of ischaemic heart disease over an 8-year study period than those with no history of chest pain.[11] 'Definite' angina was defined as chest pain brought on by exertion, situated over the sternum, forcing the person to slow down, relieved by rest and disappearing within minutes. 'Possible' angina was defined as chest pain brought on by exertion but not satisfying all the additional criteria.

A study by Schofield *et al.* reported that 10–20% of patients referred for coronary angiography because of chest pain were found to have normal coronary arteries.[12] In a series of 63 such patients they found that the only feature of chest pain to distinguish oesophageal abnormality from myocardial ischaemia was the radiation through to the back of oesophageal pain.

In addition to the immediate clinical history, factors from the patient's general history may act as a pointer to the likelihood of a positive diagnosis. Previous personal or family history of coronary heart disease, ethnic origin,[13] gender, smoking, blood pressure, hyperlipidaemia and diabetes mellitus are all relevant risk factors[14] (see pages 5–6).

In contrast, a study of survivors of sudden ischaemic near death occurring during sporting activity found no relationship between the number of risk factors and the extent of coronary arterial disease on coronary angiography.[15] In these cases the coronary event is most likely to be rupture of an atheromatous plaque induced by exercise. Similar postmortem findings were identified in 95% of patients with unstable angina and acute myocardial infarction who died suddenly. From such studies it is clear that there must be a dynamic and unpredictable element involved in coronary arterial disease.

The importance of a full history is demonstrated by a recent professional indemnity case. A 41-year-old man presented in general practice with chest pains seemingly characteristic of dyspepsia, but on subsequent delayed admission to hospital was found to have suffered a myocardial infarct and bypass surgery was later performed. The case notes revealed a history of familial hyperlipidaemia and a strong family history of ischaemic heart disease. The delay in referral and incorrect diagnosis was regarded as being of doubtful defensibility and the patient received an out-of-court settlement.[8]

The diagnosis of coronary heart disease may therefore be fraught with difficulty. Patients and general practitioners both know that angina may portend a potentially lethal condition, the outcome of which may be altered by earlier management decisions.

Expectations of patients and doctors in general practice

Many factors affect the outcome of consultations in general practice for suspected angina. These include the attitudes and expectations of both patient and doctor, the type of practice, the facilities of the local hospital, the geographical situation and, more controversially perhaps, whether the practice is fundholding. To use a computer analogy, the hardware includes the practice system and the referral system. The software variables include the patients, their relatives and the general practitioner's knowledge and confidence.

'Hardware' variables: general practice and the hospital

The electrocardiogram. Positive ischaemic findings on an ECG, although rarely seen, can help a great deal in elucidating the cause of chest pains in general practice. A study in 1989 showed that only 28% of general practitioners had access to electrocardiography during surgery hours, and only 16% outside these hours.[16] Of course, whether or not an ECG performed 'as a routine' for chest pains in the surgery is of any real benefit is another question. It has been suggested that all patients over the age of 50 with chest pain should have an electrocardiographic assessment, and that the accident and emergency department is the most appropriate place for this to occur.[17] One would have to ask the critical question as to how often ECGs change the clinical management of angina.

Modern electronic communication of ECGs via fax or cellnet[30] may provide a useful instrument for both isolated and suburban general practitioners. An ECG recorded in the practice is sent directly to a cardiac centre for either immediate or later reporting by a more experienced person. Clues can also be obtained from automated ECG reporting, although the sensitivity of such machines tends to produce false positive results.

The local hospital. A hospital which is nearby, well organised and sympathetic to the general practitioner will expedite the process of referral of cases of suspected angina whether it be for urgent assessment or for later investigation of an uncertain history. Practices in isolated geographical areas such as occur in Scotland or the North of England tend to develop their own expertise for dealing with acute chest pain out of necessity, but they are at an obvious disadvantage when wishing to refer a patient for assessment of suspected angina. Their district general hospitals may be many miles from a cardiology unit, hence the importance of consultants 'with an interest' based in peripheral hospitals.

General practitioners need to have reasonable access to a consultant with an interest in cardiology, and access also to exercise testing, preferably at a local district general hospital, in the knowledge that appropriate referral to a cardiologist for further evaluation will not be unreasonably constrained by budgetary factors consequent on the NHS reforms.

'Software' variables: the people

The doctor. General practitioners are all different. Their levels of education, personal experience and expectations will interact to determine whether or not their patients with chest pain are referred, and to whom.

The patient. Obvious clinical factors such as the site, radiation and severity of chest pain are the primary reasons for referral, but other factors are also relevant. A family history of coronary disease, a history of smoking and comorbidities such as diabetes mellitus will all influence a doctor's decision to refer. Race is also a factor; Asian men have a higher risk of myocardial infarction than white men, who in turn have a higher risk than Afro-Caribbean men.[13] Patients who are well educated, or maybe privately insured, tend to be more aware of the range of expertise available to assess and treat their condition. Some patients have relatives who advocate on their behalf, which may influence the general practitioner's actions.

Hospital staff. Good relationships between doctors in hospital and general practice are of great benefit to patients and indeed to doctors. Knowing a key member of hospital staff personally, whether it be a receptionist or the professor, may determine the course of a patient's hospital experience. However, such human factors, although important, should be no substitute for a more formal fail-safe system in which objective criteria determine the outcome of referral to hospital.

Investigation by the general practitioner before referral

A general practitioner has expectations of a referral service for patients with suspected angina, and also has obligations before referral.

A complete history should be taken and an examination performed. Both should include questions and observations that might support other diagnoses such as gall bladder disease, dyspepsia, musculoskeletal disorders such as costochondritis, cardiovascular disorders such as aortic dissection or pericarditis, or pulmonary disorders such as pleurisy. Even if the history strongly supports a diagnosis of angina, it is important to remember that angina may also result from pathology other than coronary atheroma, such as in aortic stenosis or hypertension, an increase in cardiac output as in anaemia or hyperthyroidism, or hypoxia as in chronic lung disease. In order to make outpatient appointments more efficient, a general practitioner may decide to arrange from his practice appropriate blood tests such as full blood count, thyroid function, serum lipid estimation and blood sugar; a 12-lead ECG is also useful.

Reasons for referral of suspected angina

We need to consider more closely the reasons why a patient might be referred for a secondary assessment of suspected angina for the primary case setting.

The reasons for referral lie in a combination of factors originating from both patient and doctor (Fig. 1). Some patients whose angina is progressing rapidly will be admitted as an emergency for monitoring in a coronary care unit; others in this group of unsta-

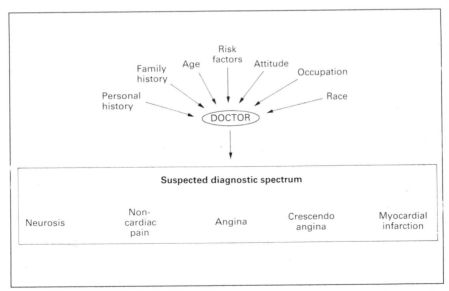

Fig. 1. *Patient factors affecting diagnostic outcome of consultation for chest pain.*

ble or crescendo angina will be managed by the general practitioner at home with drug therapy and rest prior to urgent outpatient
assessment by a consultant, probably within the working week. In
one study of some 2,000 patients who had a myocardial infarction,
20% of those who survived complained of worsening or new angina in the days or weeks before their attack.[18] Many had other symptoms such as unusual tiredness, breathlessness, indigestion or
vague chest pains. Mulcahy *et al.* suggested that there was little evidence to show that aggressive or intensive medical or surgical treatment was superior to a conservative symptomatic approach in a
coronary care unit.[19] This view is now outmoded, as has been
demonstrated by studies employing aspirin[20,32] and early thrombolysis.[21] Inpatient admission for intravenous heparin and aspirin has
been shown to reduce the infarct rate by more than 70% in
patients diagnosed as having unstable angina.

The practitioner or the patient, or both, may be uncertain about
the diagnosis. Often the doctor is able to feel satisfied that the
source of the pain is not cardiac, but the patient, suffering from
stress disorder and having experienced chest pain, is not convinced and develops a 'cardiac neurosis'. In this situation a negative stress test, when pushed to the limit, may have remarkable
therapeutic effect. A patient with established angina, but whose
confidence is lacking, may equally be reassured by a stress test that
demonstrates greater than anticipated work capacity, thereby
extending the patient's anticipated pain barrier.

From time to time, doctors will see patients with chest pain in
whom they suspect a cardiac cause but are unable to distinguish
the pain from one of non-cardiac origin by the history and presentation alone.[7] Exercise testing may be useful in these circumstances, as outlined in Chapter 5 which also explores a structured
assessment of the patient with angina.

Bennett and Atkinson prospectively studied 170 patients who
presented to hospital with chest pain, and found that general practitioners correctly diagnosed 64% of cases (emergency and outpatients).[22] Significantly, 23% of patients admitted with chest pain
were found to have alimentary tract disease only. The study
demonstrated that the clinical features of oesophageal pain may
closely resemble those of cardiac pain, with identical radiation and
precipitation by exercise and emotion. It is interesting to compare[23] these data with those from a study by Frank, a general practitioner, of 450 consecutive patients presenting with chest pain over
a 4-year period.[6] His diagnoses were made in general practice but
reviewed by a cardiologist (Fig. 2).

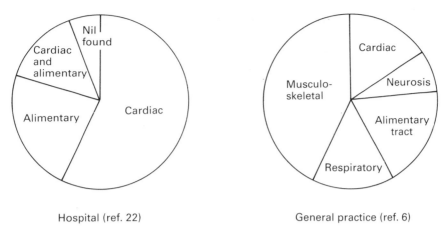

Hospital (ref. 22)   General practice (ref. 6)

Fig. 2. *Causes of pain in patients presenting in hospital and general practice.*[23]

A major problem for most general practitioners is in the group with less severe chest pain ('suspected angina') whose condition seems to be well controlled on medical treatment. Studies have shown that severity of angina is unreliable as a measure of underlying severity of coronary artery disease. A patient describing bouts of severe pain related to severe exertion may be less at risk than a patient with mild pain of increasing frequency. It is the change in pattern that is critical.

As Chapter 7 outlines, there is evidence that patients with multivessel coronary arterial disease or left main stem disease have improved survival after coronary bypass grafting,[24,25] although angina frequently recurs. Unfortunately, there is not yet a recognised and generally used method for detecting these important subgroups. How can we best select those patients at most risk for referral to a cardiologist? Regrettably, one of the most confusing aspects of this whole issue for general practitioners is the inconsistent handling of different patients with suspected angina by different consultants or departments.

Table 2 shows an attempt to outline appropriate reasons for referral. As a basis for audit, local general practitioners and cardiologists might agree on waiting times that should not be exceeded by, for example, 90% of patients in each category.

Conclusion

After a full history, examination, appropriate tests and having taken into account the patient's personal history, social circumstances and cardiovascular risk factors,[26] the general practitioner should be able

Table 2. Appropriate indications for referral from primary care.

1. Patients with unstable or crescendo angina
2. Patients with known angina whose symptom profile is altering for the worse
3. Patients with chest pain of uncertain origin (suspected angina)
4. Patients with established angina whose lack of confidence is inhibiting a normal lifestyle
5. Patients with probable non-cardiac chest pain who require reassurance over and above that which can be given by the general practitioner
6. Some patients with chest pain (probable angina) satisfactorily controlled on medication. It is this group that causes most concern since it is clinically impossible to tell if such patients have, for example, left main stem disease, for which operation is indicated.

to make an informed decision about referral (see Table 2).

Uniform questionnaires would ensure a standardised data set which would provide a degree of objectivity in referrals. In addition, such a tool would lend itself to audit,[27] not only for research and quality standards in general practice,[28,29] but also for the centre receiving the referral (eg waiting list times by referral category). Patients referred with an appropriate complete range of preliminary investigations might benefit from cheaper outpatient charges.

I particularly stress the importance of good communication, as does Michael Joy in Chapter 9. In addition, I should like to see wider based deployment of a fax-based ECG reporting service,[30] with the opportunity for immediate or same day reporting.

There are other aspects of communication. Research has shown that the factors valued most by general practitioners in a referral system include:[31]

- Availability of notes at consultation in outpatient clinics
- Respect for general practitioners in telephone conversations with hospital colleagues
- Adequate supply of medicines at discharge
- Patient management plans for general practitioners
- Early arrival of legibly signed discharge slips
- Type of doctor who sees the patient in new outpatients
- Absence of unnecessary duplication of investigations[28]

Above all, general practitioners need to know what is happening to their patients. Any practitioner is at a great disadvantage if he or she appears ignorant of the latest development in the patient's treatment processes, especially if all is not proceeding smoothly.

References

1. Royal College of General Practitioners, Office of Population Census-es and Surveys, Department of Health and Social Security. *Morbidity statistics from general practice 1981–82: third national study.* London: HMSO, 1986.
2. Office of Health Economics. *Coronary heart disease: the need for action.* London: Office of Health Economics, 1987.
3. Fry J. *Common diseases: their nature, incidence and care,* 4th edn. Lancaster: MTP Press, 1985.
4. Hodgkin K. *Towards earlier diagnosis in primary care,* 5th edn. Edinburgh: Churchill Livingstone, 1985.
5. Tunstall-Pedoe H. Angina pectoris: epidemiology and risk factors. *European Heart Journal* 1985; **6**(suppl. F): 1–5.
6. Frank PI. *Anterior chest pain in family practice.* MD thesis. University of Liverpool, 1970.
7. Master AM. The spectrum of anginal and noncardiac chest pain. *Journal of the American Medical Association* 1964; **187**: 894–9.
8. Medical Protection Society. Indigestion or infarct? *MPS General Practice Casebook* 1993; **2**: 24.
9. Rose GA. The diagnosis of ischaemic heart pain and intermittent claudication in field surveys. *Bulletin of the World Health Organization* 1962; **27**: 645–8.
10. Shaper AG, Cook DG, Walker M, Macfarlane PW. Prevalence of ischaemic heart disease in middle aged British men. *British Heart Journal* 1984; **5**: 595–605.
11. Cook DG, Shaper AG, Macfarlane PW. Using the WHO (Rose) angina questionnaire in cardiovascular epidemiology. *International Journal of Epidemiology* 1989; **18**: 607–13.
12. Schofield PM, Whorwell PJ, Jones PE, Brooks NH, Bennett DH. Differentiation of 'esophageal' and 'cardiac' chest pain. *American Journal of Cardiology* 1988; **62**: 315–6.
13. Tunstall-Pedoe H, Clayton D, Morris JN, Brigden W, McDonald L. Coronary attacks in East London. *Lancet* 1975; **ii**: 833–8.
14. American Heart Association. *Coronary risk handbook: estimating risk of coronary heart disease in daily practice.* New York: American Heart Association, 1973.
15. Ciampricotti R, el-Gamal M, Relik T *et al.* Clinical characteristics and coronary angiographic findings of patients with unstable angina, acute myocardial infarction, and survivors of sudden ischaemic death occurring during and after sport. *American Heart Journal* 1990; **120**(1): 1267–78.
16. Colquhoun MC. General practitioners' use of electrocardiography: relevance to early thrombolytic treatment. *British Medical Journal* 1989; **299**: 433.
17. Tachakra SS, Pawsey S, Beckett M, Potts D, Idowu A. Outcome of patients with chest pain discharged from an accident and emergency department. *British Medical Journal* 1991; **302**: 504–5.
18. Colling A, Dellipiani AW, Donaldson RJ, MacCormack P. Teeside coronary survey: an epidemiological study of acute attacks of myocardial infarction. *British Medical Journal* 1976; **2**: 1169–72.

19. Mulcahy R, Daly L, Graham I *et al.* Unstable angina: natural history and determinants of prognosis. *American Journal of Cardiology* 1981; **48**: 525–8.
20. Lewis HD Jr, Davis JW, Archibald DG *et al.* Protective effects of aspirin against acute myocardial infarction and death in men with unstable angina. Results of a Veterans Administration Cooperative Study. *New England Journal of Medicine* 1983; **309**: 396–403.
21. Gruppo Italiano per lo Studio della Streptochinasi nell'Infarto Miocardico (GISSI). Effectiveness of intravenous thrombolytic treatment in acute myocardial infarction. *Lancet* 1986; **i**: 397–401.
22. Bennett JR, Atkinson M. The differentiation between oesophageal and cardiac pain. *Lancet* 1966; **ii**: 1123–7.
23. Cormack JJC, Marinker M, Morrell D, eds. *Clinical management in general practice*, 2nd edn. London: Kluwer Medical, 1987.
24. Veterans Administration Coronary Artery Bypass Surgery Cooperative Study Group. Eleven years survival in the Veterans Administration randomised trial of coronary bypass surgery for stable angina. *New England Journal of Medicine* 1984; **311**: 1333–9.
25. European Coronary Surgery Study Group. Long term results of prospective randomised study of coronary artery bypass surgery in stable angina pectoris. *Lancet* 1982; **ii**: 1173–80.
26. Tunstall-Pedoe H. The Dundee coronary risk-disk for management of change in risk factors. *British Medical Journal* 1991; **303**: 744–7.
27. Ellis BW, Sensky T. A clinician's guide to setting up audit. *British Medical Journal* 1991; **302**: 704–7.
28. Grol R. National standard setting for quality of care in general practice: attitude of general practitioners and response to a set of standards. *British Journal of General Practice* 1990; **40**: 361–4.
29. O'Dowd TC, Wilson AD. Set menus and clinical freedom. *British Medical Journal* 1991; **303**: 450–2.
30. Chambers JA, Marshall AJ. Cellphone ECG transmission. *Cardiology in Practice* July/August 1991: 19–20.
31. Bowling A, Jacobsen B, Southgate L, Formby J. General practitioners' views on quality specifications for 'outpatient referrals and care contracts'. *British Medical Journal* 1991; **303**: 292–4.
32. Thévoux P, Waters D, Lam J, Jinfau M, McCans J. Reactivation of unstable angina after the discontinuation of heparin. *New England Journal of Medicine* 1992; **327**: 141–5.

5 | Structured assessment of patients with symptomatic angina pectoris in general practice and in hospital

John Irving
Consultant Physician, St John's Hospital at Howden,
Livingston, West Lothian

In this chapter, I consider the diagnosis of angina pectoris, the general assessment of the patient, and a structured approach to investigation and management. General practitioners and cardiologists share the management of patients with angina.

Diagnosis of angina pectoris

Angina pectoris is a clinical diagnosis, made on the basis of the history. This simple statement needs emphasising as patients and many physicians believe that 'tests must be done to confirm the diagnosis'.

The ability to diagnose angina only comes from experience in outpatient clinics. This experience may be limited if policies that require all new patients to be seen by a consultant are fully implemented, as young doctors in training may have less opportunities for exploring variations in the patients' histories. A number of diagnostic myths do interfere with assessment, eg that chest discomfort relieved by glyceryl trinitrate is always cardiac in origin or that chest tightness relieved by passing wind is not cardiac! Sometimes there is genuine difficulty if the doctor is not able to obtain a clear history. A second opinion is helpful. Many general practitioners are reluctant to ask simply for a 'clinical opinion', often requesting an exercise test or angiography. Community studies have found a high prevalence of symptoms suggestive of angina, particularly in women. General practitioners are therefore faced with a difficult dilemma. Do they refer everyone with chest pain to hospital? This was done in the chest pain clinic study in Edinburgh in the early 1970s.[1] A very low rate of diagnosis of angina was found amongst the referred patients in this study; in addition, on follow-up there was a relatively low rate of development of infarction or further complications.

Exercise tests

Referral letters to cardiology clinics frequently request 'confirmation of the diagnosis of angina pectoris by exercise testing'. Official bodies, such as the Department of Transport, make statements that ischaemic heart disease 'confirmed by exercise test' may be a bar to holding a vocational licence. Is such diagnostic confidence justified? That many physicians consider an exercise test as a diagnostic procedure is confirmed in a recent survey of Scottish hospitals carried out by Dr Rodger and myself. There has been a marked increase in the number of exercise tests done over the past five years to a total of approximately 22,000 per year. The indication to undertake the test is very frequently for the diagnosis of chest pain. Much of this chapter evaluates the role of exercise testing in patients with chest pain.

When an experienced clinician makes a diagnosis of angina pectoris, coronary arteriography is likely to demonstrate significant disease in 85–90% of patients. One example illustrating this point comes from the coronary artery surgery study (CASS) in the United States.[2] Table 1 shows that patients entered into the trial would have coronary artery disease more reliably detected by the history alone than by the exercise test. When the history was atypical, exercise testing did not enhance the diagnostic accuracy. This large trial demonstrates the limitations of the exercise test, admittedly among a highly selected group of individuals attending major referral centres in the United States. Such studies may not always be relevant to the community, as patients only entered the trial after other causes of angina, such as aortic stenosis or other features, had been excluded.

Exercise tests may actually give false positive results. Froelicher

Table 1. Correlation of clinical diagnosis, arteriographic evidence of coronary artery disease and exercise ECG: data from CASS in the USA.[2]

Clinical diagnosis of angina	Certain	Possible	Atypical
Arteriographic evidence of IHD	87%	66%	20%
'Positive' exercise ECG	60%	43%	20%

et al. showed that aircrew with atypical symptoms had very high rates of false positive exercise tests.[3] The CASS data also demonstrate that atypical pain is rarely associated with diagnostic exercise tests. In summary, when angina pectoris is unlikely from the history, an exercise test has a low likelihood of contributing to the diagnostic process.

When evaluating the electrocardiogram recorded during exercise, the traditional technique is to divide ST segment changes into positive or negative. There are many publications on the effects of drugs, changes in electrolyte concentration, strenuous exercise and age on ST segment changes.[4,5] Master, one of the pioneers in exercise testing, originally stated that ST depression of 1 mm or more was diagnostic of coronary disease.[6] However, the extension of exercise testing to other groups, including asymptomatic men and women, has made clear its limitations. From Bayes' theorem[7] the exercise test will be most accurate when the pre-test risk of coronary artery disease is high; for example, it is better in men than in women, and better in smokers than in non-smokers. Several groups have produced algorithms to estimate pre- and post-test probability of coronary artery disease. Morise *et al.* incorporated such pre-test variables as age, gender, diabetes, cholesterol, along with ECG variables, to produce an algorithm which was validated in other centres.[8] A more practical approach has been described in the guidelines for cardiac exercise testing recently produced for the European Society of Cardiology.[9] These guidelines use clinical variables derived from two Dutch studies to try to give greater confidence to the results of the exercise test.

In assessing the value of ST segment changes on exercise electrocardiography, many factors have to be taken together. Detry *et al.* showed that classification of patients on the basis of ST segments was the same as that based on clinical history.[10] Multivariate analysis showed that improved classification required the addition of other factors such as heart rate, onset of angina during test workload and ST segment slope. Few of us at present have access to computerised multivariate analysis, but the technology is available and is now being incorporated in some new exercise testing equipment. ST depression of 1 mm is commonly noted in middle-aged women.[11,12] Characteristically, this only occurs at high heart rates, often in the inferior leads and usually returning rapidly to normal as the tachycardia settles. The aetiology of these ST segment changes is uncertain. One speculation provoked a study of the administration of oestrogens to healthy young men. This was shown to result in the development of ST segment changes of the type described above. The frequency of such ST changes results in high false positive rates in exercise tests in women,[12] also described in asymptomatic men.[3] The low sensitivity and specificity of these tests in asymptomatic individuals allowed the pilots' trade union in the United States to prevent the introduction of compulsory annual exercise tests for all aircrew. Froelicher *et al.* had documented both high false positive and also false negative tests among aircrew obliged to undergo arteriography on the basis of abnormal ST segment changes.[3] In analysing the ST changes closely, it was found that these tended to occur in the inferior leads and at a relatively high workload. If these factors are taken into account in the interpretation of the results, there would be a reduced likelihood of false positive tests. The relationship between ST segment changes and heart rate will be emphasised later.

ST depression noted in asymptomatic men does, however, indicate a likelihood of developing clinical features of coronary artery disease at some point in the future.[13] The Seattle heart watch study suggests that this is of a similar order to a history of heavy smoking; put another way, an ischaemic exercise test is a risk factor or indicator of an increased likelihood of developing clinical disease.[14] In a different population, the kind of population frequently referred to hospital for assessment of chest pain, the risk of cardiac events in men was approximately 3% per year when ST segment depression was found. In women the risk was less than 1% per year for a positive test and 0.06% for a negative test.[15] The positive predictive value of exercise tests in such a population is clearly very low. Unfortunately patients may be wrongly informed that they have ischaemic heart disease on the basis of wrong interpretation of ST segment changes.

The clinical history may be amplified by observing the patient and recording symptoms during an exercise test. Detry *et al.* have shown that angina during the test increased the predictive value of the test. Cole and Ellestad had previously demonstrated that chest pain during the test doubled the risk of subsequent cardiac events among approximately 1,000 patients with abnormal exercise tests.[16] Hence the development of angina during the test makes the presence of coronary artery disease much more likely.

In practical terms, where a clear history linking symptoms and exercise cannot be obtained, it will rarely be helpful to undertake an exercise test. In addition, some individuals are unable to undertake an adequate exercise test, either from inability to walk on a treadmill or from associated disease.

Technical limitations in ECG recordings should now be much less. Most centres have dedicated stress-testing equipment, which partly eliminates baseline drift and reduces artifact. However, it does not negate the necessity for adequate training of technicians, for proper skin preparation and adequate lead systems. The greatest value of the exercise test relates to its potential ability to reproduce the symptoms, to observe the patient during the test, and in that sense it may be considered to be an extension of the clinical history.

General assessment of the patient

The recommendations summarised in Table 2 may be modified by age or local practice. The aim of this assessment is to determine the appropriate management options.

While most patients with angina pectoris will have coronary artery disease, the detection of aortic valve disease, hypertrophic cardiomyopathy, anaemia and so on is important. In some, associated other vascular disease, the presence of heart failure or concurrent chronic respiratory disease will strongly influence management.

Value of the resting 12 lead ECG

Many patients are falsely reassured by a normal record, or conversely made anxious by a non-specific abnormality. However, there may be helpful information. The finding of ST depression in

Table 2. Recommendations for the general medical assessment of a patient with symptomatic angina.

Clinical history
Evidence of previous myocardial infarction, other vascular disease, cardiac failure, chronic respiratory disease, history of smoking, hypertension, diabetes

Examination
Evidence of cardiac failure, valve disease, cardiac arrhythmias, other vascular disease, hypertension

12 lead ECG
Detection of ischaemia, left ventricular hypertrophy bundle branch block

Blood count
To exclude anaemia

Risk factor check
Weight, blood pressure, urinalysis, serum lipids

---

a patient with recent onset angina may be an indication to proceed directly to coronary arteriography. Hypertrophic cardiomyopathy may only be suspected from the ECG. Although the detection rate of abnormalities may be low, the 12 lead ECG clearly influences therapeutic decisions.

Risk factors

The check for risk factors may be modified by age, Fasting lipids done in 80-year-olds would not be helpful. The appropriate age limit for such screening is controversial; most physicians recommend 60–65 years. Screening for hypertension and diabetes may be useful at any age.

Modification of risk factors will be attempted by most doctors, as will the prescription of low dose aspirin–advised for most forms of vascular disease.

Other investigations

There are a number of other investigations that may be recommended, particularly in cardiac clinics. Chest X-rays may be done to detect unsuspected lung disease or heart failure, but in the absence of any clinical indication the routine use of chest X-rays in patients with angina pectoris seems unwarranted. Cardiology clinics may recommend routine echocardiography to assess left ventricular function or detect unsuspected abnormalities. No formal evaluation of these practices has been reported.

Investigation and treatment options for angina pectoris

The symptoms described by the patients are the most important influence in determining management. Mild angina, interfering rarely with activities, may be managed with prophylactic glyceryl trinitrate, aspirin and reassurance. Angina provoked by minimal exertion or at rest, particularly when of recent onset, may require immediate arteriography with a view to angioplasty. Neither of these clinical scenarios requires an exercise ECG. However, the exercise test is a useful adjunct to the history in most cases, particularly as the angiographically determined severity of coronary artery disease does not correlate with symptoms. Exercise testing should be seen as a way of stratifying risk. A patient diagnosed to have angina on clinical assessment may prove to have the exercise test. The CASS data indicate that about 20% of American patients with angina will have normal exercise tests. This does not mean that the exercise test has no relevance, but it certainly indicates that there is a good prognosis. Prognostic information from the exercise test relates to systolic pressure changes, exercise duration as well as ST segment changes. Systolic pressure and duration of exercise seem to relate to left ventricular function, whereas ST segment changes relate to extent of disease. When coronary arteriography is available, useful additional prognostic information is obtained from the exercise variables. For example, the 4-year survival for patients with symptomatic coronary disease in the CASS study ranged from 100% for those who managed stage 5 of the Bruce protocol to 53% for those who only reached the first stage. A high-risk subgroup could be defined based on the history of congestive failure, duration of exercise and/or significant ST segment depression.

In the Seattle heart watch data, factors relating to left ventricular function were more predictive of future events than any ST segment changes.[14] This relates to the high prevalence of patients with previous infarction and with impaired left ventricular function within the study population. Where patients have mild disease, the ST segment changes appear to have more value. Table 3 shows results from lipid research clinics in the United States.[17] The group had few symptoms but obviously a high *a priori* risk of coronary disease. The original reason for setting up CASS was the conflicting results from follow-up of patients with three-vessel disease. Surgical studies indicated improved prognosis in those with left main and three-vessel disease, while other studies had shown a low mortality rate on medical treatment, particularly if the exercise test was normal.[18,19] If ischaemic changes were present, the outlook was related to duration of exercise sustained during the test.

There is also a link between duration of exercise, heart rate and

Table 3. Mortality rates (per cent per year) in North American men attending lipid research clinics. Data from reference 17.

Exercise test		
	Not ischaemic	3.2
	Inconclusive	11
	Mildly ischaemic	12.6
	Strongly ischaemic	25

severity of coronary disease. The ST depression at low workload correlates closely with severe coronary disease, while ST depression only at high heart rates will not correlate; for example, healthy men exercised rapidly may reach a heart rate of 200 beats per minute with definite ST segment depression while having no evidence whatsoever of coronary artery disease.[20] The evidence from the literature therefore supports the use of the exercise ECG in stratifying the extent of coronary disease in patients with definite angina. Those with marked ST segment changes at a low workload, particularly those who have angina on the exercise test, should have arteriography and may go on to have surgery. The patient with angina but with good exercise tolerance and ST depression only at a higher heart rate could reasonably be treated medically.

The exercise test may provide other more specific information, eg ST elevation on the ECG. This is unusual but, if it develops in an individual with no prior history of myocardial infarction, it is a clear indication of a severe coronary stenosis. It is one method of selecting those individuals suitable for angioplasty. However, ST elevation may also be noted in the same leads as have demonstrated the pattern of a previous anterior infarct, and characteristically may last several minutes after exercise. This has been shown to be related to increase in wall motion abnormalities in the left ventricle.

This introduces the role of the exercise test in the patient who has had a myocardial infarction. Traditionally this is carried out either in hospital or within a month of discharge. The main value of the test is again in extending the clinical assessment with an objective measure of exercise capacity. Continued symptoms of angina after infarction, or angina induced by the exercise test, have both been shown to indicate a poor prognosis. If this is accompanied by ST depression in the ECG leads remote from the infarction, most cardiologists would recommend arteriography. ST depression in the anterior leads (so-called reciprocal ST depression in the patient with an acute inferior infarct) is another method of identifying individuals who will subsequently have an abnormal exercise test and who have a high likelihood of having three-vessel disease. However, follow-up studies have given some conflicting results. The original study from Montreal demonstrated a marked excess mortality in those with ST depression when tested ten days after infarction.[21] However, Jennings *et al.* from Newcastle found that ST changes were not predictive and that subsequent events and mortality related more to left ventricular function.[22] These differences, of course, demonstrate the importance of the definition of the population studied. The Montreal group excluded those with impaired left ventricular function, while the Newcastle group studied consecutive patients.

Interpretation of the post-infarct exercise test must take account of the site of infarction, left ventricular function and symptoms in addition to ECG changes. Satisfactory duration of exercise and a normal increase in systolic pressure will provide the most useful prognostic information. This usually correlates with complications in the early phase of the infarct, particularly pulmonary oedema. Where impaired left ventricular function is considered likely, follow-up methods would focus on the risk of congestive heart failure and assessing left ventricular function by ventriculography or cardiac ultrasound. The exercise test therefore in this group is defining those who have impaired left ventricular function.

If infarction is a non-Q-wave type, sometimes called subendocardial, the subsequent exercise test will allow selection of those requiring arteriography, possibly with angioplasty. Selection would be based on poor exercise tolerance and ST segment changes at low workload. ST segment changes may often take the form of 'normalising' deep anterior T-waves. If such an abnormal test is accompanied by symptoms, early arteriography will usually be undertaken.

Prolonged ischaemic chest pain without infarction, sometimes described as unstable angina, pre-infarction angina or acute coronary insufficiency, is a frequent cause of admission to coronary care units. Many physicians consider exercise testing to be contraindicated, at least in the acute phase, preferring to treat with beta-blockers, aspirin and nitrates. An exercise test may be undertaken in three to four weeks to determine exercise duration and any ST changes. However, prolonged ischaemic pain accompanied by transient T-wave changes will usually justify early arteriography without preliminary exercise testing.[23] To delay the exercise test for three to four weeks after the acute episode, either of infarction or unstable angina, is appropriate as in the UK invasive investigations often have a waiting list of weeks or even months, and early pre-discharge tests have poor specificity.

Conclusion

Figures 1 and 2 show two algorithms which summarise the management of the patient with angina; particular emphasis is placed on the role of the exercise test. If these guidelines were followed, facilities for 300 exercise tests per year per 100,000 population would be required.

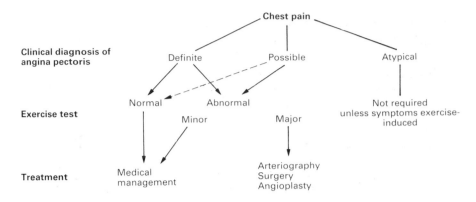

Fig. 1. *Management of chest pain.*

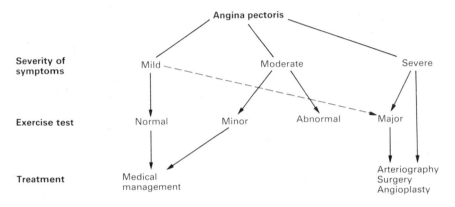

Fig. 2. *Management of angina pectoris.*

References

1. Duncan B, Fulton M, Morrison SL *et al.* Prognosis of new and worsening angina pectoris. *British Medical Journal* 1976; **i**: 981–90.
2. Weiner DA, Ryan TJ, McCabe CH *et al.* Exercise stress testing: correlations among history of angina, ST segment response and prevalence of coronary disease in CASS. *New England Journal of Medicine* 1979; **301**: 230–7.
3. Froelicher VF, Thompson AG, Wolthius R, *et al.* Angiographic findings in asymptomatic aircrewmen with electrocardiographic abnormalities. *American Journal of Cardiology* 1974; **39**: 322–40.
4. Epstein SE. Limitations of electrocardiographic exercise testing. *New England Journal of Medicine* 1979; **301**: 264–5.
5. Chung EK. *Exercise electrocardiography: practical approach*, 2nd edn. Baltimore: Williams and Wilkins, 1983.
6. Master AM. The Master two step. *American Heart Journal* 1968; **75**: 809–11.
7. Diamond GA. Reverend Bayes' silent majority. *American Journal of Cardiology* 1986; **57**: 1175–6.

8. Morise AP, Detrane R, Bobbio M, Diamond GA. Development and validation of a logistic regression-derived algorithm for estimating the incremental probability of coronary artery disease before and after exercise testing. *Journal of the American College of Cardiology* 1992; **20**: 1187–96.

9. Dargie HJ. Guildeines for cardiac exercise testing. *European Heart Journal* 1993; **14**: 969–88.

10. Detry JMR, Robert A, Luwaert RT *et al.* Diagnostic value of computerised exercise testing in men without previous myocardial infarction. *European Heart Journal* 1985; **6**: 227–38.

11. Cumming GR, Dufreme C, Kich L, Gavin T. Exercise tests in normal women. *British Heart Journal* 1973; **35**: 1055.

12. Melin JA, Wijns W, Vanbutsele RJ *et al.* Alternative diagnostic strategies for coronary artery disease in women. *Circulation* 1985; **71**: 535–42.

13. Doyle JT, Kinch SH. The prognosis of an abnormal exercise test. *Circulation* 1970; **41**: 545–52.

14. Bruce R, Di Rouen T, Peterson DR *et al.* Non-invasive predictions of sudden cardiac death in men with CHD. *American Journal of Cardiology* 1977; **39**: 833–40.

15. Manca C, Dei Caa L, Albertini D *et al.* Different prognostic value of exercise electrocardiograms in men and women. *Cardiology* 1978; **63**: 312–18.

16. Cole JP, Ellestad MH. Significance of chest pain during treadmill exercise. *American Journal of Cardiology* 1978; **41**: 227.

17. Gordon DJ, Ekelund LG, Karon JM *et al.* Predictive value of the exercise test for mortality in North American men. *Circulation* 1986; **74**: 252–60.

18. Weiner DA, Ryan TJ, McCabe *et al.* Prognostic importance of a clinical profile and exercise test in medically treated patients with coronary artery disease. *Journal of the American College of Cardiology* 1984; **3**: 772–9.

19. Dagenais GR, Rouleau JR, Christen A, Fabia J. Survival of patients with a strongly positive exercise ECG. *Circulation* 1982; **65**: 452–6.

20. Barnard RJ, MacAlpin R, Kattus AA, Buckberg CD. Ischaemic response to sudden strenuous exercise in healthy men. *Circulation* 1973; **48**: 936–41.

21. Theroux P, Waters DD, Halphen C *et al.* Prognostic value of exercise testing soon after myocardial infarction. *New England Journal of Medicine* 1979; **301**: 341–5.

22. Jennings K, Reid DS, Hawkins T, Julian DJ. Role of exercise testing early after myocardial infarction in identifying candidates for coronary surgery. *British Medical Journal* 1984; **288**: 185–7.

23. Wilson JA, Irving JB. Management of patients with prolonged ischaemic chest pain without acute myocardial infarction. *American Heart Journal* 1988; **115**: 1182–5.

6 | Coronary arteriography in the management of the patient with suspected angina

Raphael Balcon
Consultant Cardiologist
Simon Davies
Senior Registrar in Cardiology, The London Chest Hospital

Cardiac catheterisation was first performed over 60 years ago, and the first attempts at selective cannulation of the coronary arteries 40 years ago. Coronary arteriography now plays a central role in the management of patients with coronary artery disease. We shall first consider the theoretical issues in the use of coronary arteriography for diagnosis, for management, and for other purposes such as research. Following this we will list the limitations of coronary arteriography, and then discuss the indications for arteriography in stable patients and in unstable patients.

Uses of coronary arteriography

Coronary arteriography may be used in the diagnosis of coronary artery disease. Although this might seem to be a straightforward statement, there are limitations, and failure to appreciate these is the cause of much confusion and apparent diagnostic difficulty. Angina is an intermittent pathophysiological state; it cannot be diagnosed from a coronary arteriogram, which merely reveals structural coronary artery disease. Angina may occur when the coronary arteries are normal, for example in severe aortic stenosis, in intermittent coronary spasm, and in syndrome X (the syndrome of angina with objective evidence of myocardial ischaemia, eg thallium scanning, and angiographically normal coronary arteries). Conversely, the demonstration of coronary artery disease does not prove that a patient's symptoms are caused by intermittent myocardial ischaemia. In practice, coronary arteriography is rarely needed for *diagnosis,* and proper clinical assessment is preferable. It may be necessary in patients with atypical symptoms and/or equivocal results of non-invasive testing who are young, or particularly anxious, or in certain occupational groups such as aeroplane pilots or those who drive heavy goods vehicles (in the UK, HGV Class 1).*

Coronary arteriography is most useful in guiding the management of patients with angina. In general terms, the aims of treatment of angina are to alleviate symptoms and to improve prognosis. It is the latter that gives rise to difficulty. The use of coronary arteriography in patients with severe angina, despite optimal medical therapy, to assess their suitability for coronary artery bypass graft (CABG) or percutaneous coronary angiography (PTCA) to improve their angina presents no problems. However, the observation that CABG improves prognosis of certain groups of patients with coronary artery disease even if they have few symptoms suggests that more patients with milder angina should be considered for arteriography. In these patients, coronary arteriography guides treatment in two ways:

- Assessing prognosis from the extent of coronary disease, so as to select patients expected to obtain improved survival after intervention
- Selection of the appropriate intervention (CABG or PTCA)

Left ventricular function is also assessed at the time of coronary arteriography, and this may influence selection for intervention. There is also an opportunity to assess coincidental disease of the cardiac valves, great vessels and lungs, although all of these can usually be assessed with other techniques.

Coronary ateriography is employed in a variety of research settings. These include studies of coronary vasomotor control and peptides, angiographic follow-up of restenosis after PTCA, and angiographic follow-up of lipid-lowering agents. Other than atherosclerotic disease, coronary arteriography may diagnose rare conditions such as Kawasaki disease (mucocutaneous lymph node syndrome), anomalous coronary arteries, and define the arterial supply of the exceptionally rare primary cardiac tumours.

Limitations of coronary arteriography

The most obvious limitations of coronary arteriography are the practical problems of the cost and the small but definite risk

---

*Since April 1993 vocational licensing for motor vehicles in the UK has depended on the unmedicated patient reaching the end of Stage III of the Bruce protocol exercise test without major symptoms or haemodynamic problems. Angiography is no longer specified.

(mortality less than 1 per 1,000). Linked to cost is the limited availability of coronary arteriography, especially in the UK.

Angina is a pathophysiological state with a number of potential contributory mechanisms, including coronary spasm, variation in microvascular resistance and coronary flow reserve and in collateral supply, which may not be visible on arteriography until normal perfusion is reduced.

A coronary arteriogram provides a single *snapshot* of the state of the coronary arteries and provides a structural rather than a functional assessment. It cannot account for variation in susceptibility to ischaemic damage (cellular conditioning) or in the threshold of perception of pain or discomfort.

Coronary arteriography only identifies disease of the arterial walls that impinges on the lumen, causing stenosis or ectasia. Histopathological studies show that extensive coronary atheroma may be present in arteries that are angiographically normal.

Some of these limitations might in theory be addressed by extending the arteriographic procedure to include provocation with ergonovine to assess spasm, detailed analysis of lesion morphology, calculation of angiographic coronary risk scores, digital imaging analysis of coronary flow, flow analysis with Doppler ultrasound tipped catheters, and cross-sectional imaging of the coronary wall with intravascular ultrasound. However, none of these has yet justified the additional time, cost or risks in routine practice.

In addition to these limitations, there are limitations due to interpretation and analysis of the results of coronary angiography. Experimental data have shown that maximal coronary flow is limited by a stenosis of approximately 30% of the diameter and resting flow by one of 90%. It is conventional to regard as significant lesions that cause 70% or more stenosis of diameter, which equates to approximately 50% reduction in cross-sectional area. However, the resistance of a lesion also depends on other factors such as length; multiple lesions in series have a complex effect on flow reduction. The problem is compounded by the often unknown and variable effect of collateral flow.

Deciding the location and severity of stenoses may be difficult even for experienced observers when there is foreshortening of the image, and overlap of the coronary segments in different views. This, together with the potential bias introduced by knowledge of other clinical factors, may be responsible for intra- and inter-observer variation in grading stenoses. These problems can be overcome to a certain extent by *blind* assessment, although this is not practicable in routine clinical work. It is, however, essential for research purposes when accurate measurements are made using callipers or by computer. Computer-based measurements, perhaps not surprisingly, introduced new problems, particularly because there were systematic differences between the computed result and visual grading.

A final difficulty is that coronary lesions progress in a variable, intermittent and unpredictable manner. Myocardial infarction may occur on the basis of an event such as rupture of a minor atheromatous plaque.

It is perhaps surprising therefore that the 'snapshot' of arteriography is as good as it is at predicting outcome. It is the standard clinical method and has been used in most studies relating prognosis to extent of disease. It was the method employed by the three major trials of coronary surgery accepted as the standards for current practice.[1-3]

Prognostic significance of coronary arteriography and the selection of patients for coronary artery surgery

The prognostic significance of coronary arteriography was well demonstrated in the early 1970s using visually assessed coronary angiograms. The number of major coronary arteries affected by a stenosis of 50% or more, and the amount of left ventricular damage, were shown to predict the subsequent survival (Fig. 1).

A number of workers attempted to improve the predictive value of coronary arteriography by devising coronary scores to assess the proportion of myocardium at risk, which it was hoped would correlate even better with prognosis.

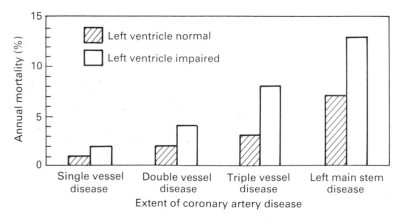

Fig. 1. *Annual mortality in coronary artery disease.*

Figure 2 shows the 5-year survival of patients classified according to the Coronary Index[4] and according to the standard categories. Although in each there is the expected relationship between disease severity and survival, the detailed Coronary Index adds little to the discrimination of high risk and low risk groups. No other index yielded any more information and none is in routine clinical use.

In the late 1970s and early 1980s the three large randomised trials compared survival after elective coronary bypass surgery with that following medical therapy.[1-3] Some controversy continues as to the exact interpretation of the results, but there was improved survival after surgery in groups with more than 50% stenosis of the left main stem or with severe proximal triple vessel disease. In the ECSSG study there was also improved survival with surgery in patients with double vessel disease, if one of the affected vessels was the LAD, with impaired left ventricular function.[3]

Indications for coronary arteriography

With these considerations in mind, appropriate indications for coronary arteriography are now summarised:

- Diagnosis of the cause of chest pain in a few selected cases (discussed above)
- Planning coronary intervention (CABG or PTCA) in patients with angina not controlled with optimal medical therapy, either not responding satisfactorily to maximal therapy or unable to tolerate drugs that are normally effective.
- Patients whose angina is satisfactorily controlled with medical

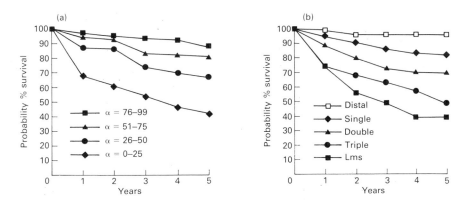

Fig. 2. *Five-year survival of patients according to two classifications of the arteriographic extent of coronary artery disease.* (a) *The Coronary Index.* (b) *Standard clinical classification.*

therapy, but who might obtain improved survival from intervention, ie those patients in whom there is sufficient probability that coronary arteriography would identify triple vessel or left main stem disease with prognostic benefit from elective CABG; this includes patients following myocardial infarction. The operation improves survival in these groups, irrespective of severity of symptoms (and probably even in those without symptoms). Unfortunately the correlation between extent of coronary disease and level of angina is weak, so symptoms are a poor predictor of those patients who might benefit from CABG. The correlation between the results of non-invasive testing such as exercise testing (Chapter 5) and the extent of coronary disease is also imprecise, and may not be sufficient to detect all those patients who might have prognostic benefit from CABG.

Given these premises, the logical conclusion would be that all patients with angina should undergo coronary arteriography so as to identify all cases whose life expectancy would be improved by surgery. This is clearly not practicable in terms of resources, and with large numbers of low risk patients the dangers of coronary arteriography become significant compared with the probability of benefit. The practical definition of 'those patients in whom there is sufficient probability that coronary arteriography would identify triple vessel or left main stem disease with prognostic benefit from elective CABG' is, in the present state of knowledge, a matter of opinion. It probably includes patients with angina (even if well controlled) whose exercise test is strongly abnormal at a low workload.

The following are the best guidelines for arteriography that can at present be given:

• Patients undergoing cardiac catheterisation for other types of cardiac disease with a view to cardiac surgery, who have chest pains or definite angina, or who are of an age at which coronary disease is common (say, men over 50 years and women over 60 years)

• Patients with unstable angina
  (a) who have continuing symptoms — either definite, with ECG changes, or possible, with undiagnosed episodes of chest pain at rest
  (b) who have settled with medical therapy. Two policies prevail. In the first, arteriography is advised for all patients after unstable angina, irrespective of other factors, as the

probability of further coronary events is high. Alternatively, arteriography is advised only for those patients at especially high risk. Risk factors include: an antecedent history of angina; previous myocardial infarction; an exercise test after settling on medical therapy which is strongly abnormal at a low workload; and a few patients in whom the diagnosis of their chest pain remains uncertain.

The first policy is preferred but, where facilities for coronary arteriography are severely limited, the second may be unavoidable.

Contraindications to coronary arteriography

In practice contraindications are few. Other major diseases that influence survival and considerably increase the risks of

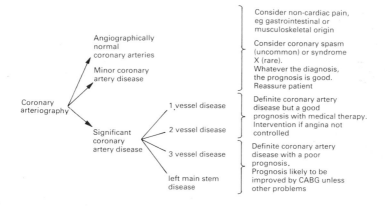

Fig. 3. *Management of coronary disease.*

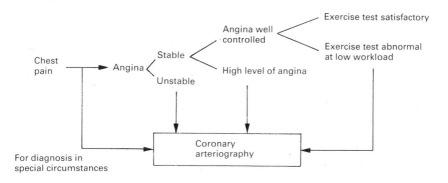

Fig. 4. *Management of coronary disease: simplified scheme.*

intervention are a relative contraindication, although severe persistent symptoms may demand taking the risk. Problems such as uncontrolled heart failure, uncontrolled hypertension, hypokalaemia and/or digitalis toxicity or excessive anticoagulation are best dealt with before angiography. Allergy to radiographic contrast media can usually be overcome by pretreatment with antihistamines and steroids.

Conclusions

There is no doubt that knowledge of the coronary anatomy greatly aids the management of patients with suspected angina (Fig. 3). In practice, the problem is to select those patients who will benefit most, given limited resources. A greatly simplified scheme is given in Fig. 4.

Advances in PTCA add a further dimension to the problem: many patients who might not be considered for CABG because of relatively mild symptoms or because of severe co-existing medical problems are now having coronary arteriography with a view to angioplasty.

References

1. CASS principal investigators and their associates. Coronary artery surgery study (CASS): a randomised trial of coronary artery bypass surgery. Survival data. *Circulation* 1983; **68**: 939–50.
2. European coronary surgery study group. Long-term results of prospective randomised study of coronary artery bypass surgery in stable angina pectoris. *Lancet* 1982; **ii**: 1173–80.
3. Veterans Administration Coronary Artery Bypass Surgery Cooperative Study Group. Eleven-year survivors in the Veterans Administration randomised trial of coronary bypass surgery for stable angina. *New England Journal of Medicine* 1984; **311**: 1333.
4. Balcon R. Prognostic significance of coronary arteriography. *Acta Medica Portuguesa* 1980; Suppl 1:9: 9–15.

7 | What can cardiac intervention achieve?

David de Bono

Professor of Cardiology, University of Leicester

This chapter reviews outcomes after coronary angioplasty (PTCA) or bypass grafting (CABG). It is useful to distinguish between technical outcomes, for example, restenosis rates in angioplasty or graft patency in bypass grafting, and clinical outcomes such as survival, freedom from symptoms and quality of life.

Technical outcomes

Approximately 70% of saphenous vein bypass grafts have become occluded after ten years. Patency rates after this interval are slightly higher for internal mammary artery grafts.[1] Aspirin plus dipyridamole has been shown to improve early saphenous vein graft patency,[2] but no agent has been shown to affect late patency rates. Using angiographic criteria, approximately 30% of segments dilated at angioplasty will become restenosed, most of them within the first three months after angioplasty. The restenosis rate for repeat angioplasty is similar to that for primary angioplasty.[3]

Clinical outcomes

Clinical outcomes correlate poorly with technical outcomes. Patients with late graft occlusion may not suffer clinical angina because a collateral circulation has developed, or because advancing age reduces physical activity. Neither recurrent symptoms nor a 'positive' exercise test alone are reliable predictors of post-angioplasty restenosis; the combination is specific but not very sensitive. Despite the enormous number of procedures, reliable outcome data come from only a restricted number of studies, frequently involving selected patient groups. Mortality data are generally reliable but provide only a fragment of clinically useful information. Quality of life measures are affected by a placebo effect associated with either procedure, and from lack of standardisation of instruments. Data about return to work are of economic interest, but vary with the economic state of the nation and the social status of the patient.

Outcome after coronary bypass surgery

The main sources of reliable data for the effects of coronary bypass grafting in stable angina are the European CAST (Coronary Artery Surgery Trial)[4] and North American CASS (Coronary Artery Surgery Study) trials.[5-7] Both trials randomised patients between bypass grafting and medical treatment, both recruited patients with at least some symptoms of angina, and both showed a survival advantage of surgical over medical treatment in patients with left main coronary stenosis, three-vessel coronary disease (especially if associated with impaired left ventricular function), and specific types of two-vessel disease. There was no survival advantage in single-vessel disease. Patients with multivessel disease but good exercise tolerance did well with or without surgery.

In patients entered in the CASS registry with three-vessel disease and class 1–2 angina at presentation, 5-year survival was 90% in the surgically treated and 72% in the medically treated group.[4] Patients with class 3–4 angina had an 87% chance of survival at five years with surgery, and 59% with medical treatment.[5]

It must be remembered that the results of these trials may not be entirely applicable to everyday practice. At least 50%, and frequently a higher proportion, of patients considered for these randomised trials were considered to be so severe, or their coronary anatomy so unfavourable, that randomisation would be inappropriate. Follow-up of such patients has been reported in a number of open studies.

In general, coronary bypass surgery is associated with an operative mortality of less than 1%, and 80% of patients are free from anginal symptoms at one year. 'Return to work' rates vary from 20% to 80% depending on the study.[8] Apart from specifically surgical complications such as wound infection, minor neurological disturbance is common but nearly always self-limiting.[9] Wound pain and musculoskeletal pain relating to the sternotomy incision occur to some extent in nearly all patients, but usually subside spontaneously. Those patients who return to work usually do so about three months after the operation.

The joint American College of Cardiology/American Heart Association task force have attempted to summarise the complex issues surrounding coronary bypass surgery by defining three classes of indication:[10]

I.   Conditions for which the operation is indicated on the basis of a demonstrated advantage over medical treatment in terms of longevity, relief of symptoms, or both

II.   Conditions for which the operation is acceptable treatment but for which its advantages over medical treatment have not yet been fully defined

III. Conditions for which the operation is not generally considered to be indicated because of lack of demonstrated advantage over medical treatment.

It is also necessary to consider the class of angina (Table 1).

The effects of ventricular function and angiographic findings on the treatment class of patients with chronic stable class 3 or 4 angina are shown in Table 2. The presence or absence of ischaemia on non-invasive stress testing has been claimed not to affect the treatment class, but this is simply because very few, if any, patients with class 3 or 4 angina have a negative stress test.

Table 1. Canadian Cardiovascular Society functional classification.

Class 1. Ordinary physical activity, such as walking and climbing stairs, does not cause angina. Angina with strenuous or rapid or prolonged exertion at work or recreation.

Class 2. Slight limitation of ordinary activity. Angina with walking or climbing stairs rapidly, walking uphill, walking or stair climbing after meals, in cold, in wind, or when under emotional stress, or only during the few hours after awakening. Angina with walking more than two blocks on the level and climbing more than one flight of ordinary stairs at a normal pace and in normal conditions.

Class 3. Marked limitation of ordinary physical activity. Angina with walking one to two blocks on the level and climbing more than one flight in normal conditions.

Class 4. Inability to carry on any physical activity without discomfort. Anginal syndrome may be present at rest.

Table 2. Treatment class of patients with class 3 or 4 angina and different degrees of left ventricular dysfunction.

	Left ventricular dysfunction			
	None	Mild	Moderate	Severe
Left main	I	I	I	I
3 vessel	I	I	I	I
2 vessel	II	II	II	II
1 vessel	II	II	II	II

Patients with *unstable angina* have been shown in the short term to fare equally well with medical or surgical treatment on an intention to treat basis, but this is to some extent a selection artifact, as patients with persistent symptoms select themselves for surgery. A previous history of unstable angina makes elective bypass grafting more attractive.

Outcome after coronary angioplasty

Controlled data about angioplasty outcome are scanty. Parisi and colleagues randomised 212 patients (out of a potential population of 9,573) to angioplasty or to continued medical management.[11] At six months, relief of angina and objective exercise tolerance was somewhat better in the angioplasty group, at the cost of an increased risk of myocardial infarction or bypass grafting. Angioplasty for chronic stable angina has an operative mortality rate of less than 1%, and a myocardial infarct/emergency surgery rate of 3–8%.[8]

The RITA (Randomised Intervention Treatment of Angina) trial is a recent United Kingdom trial which has attempted to compare outcomes in patients randomised to treatment either with coronary bypass grafting or with coronary angioplasty.[12] An important entrance criterion was that both angioplaster and surgeon should agree that they could achieve the same level of revascularisation. One thousand and eleven patients were randomised (approximately 3% of those undergoing angiography at the participating units). Fifty nine per cent had grade 3 or 4 angina, and 55% had two or more diseased vessels. After a mean follow-up period of 2.5 years, overall mortality was 3.4% and was similar in the angioplasty and bypass graft groups. Death or non-fatal myocardial infarction occurred in 9.2% of patients, and again there was no difference between the groups. There was considerable symptomatic relief of angina in both groups, with an average increase in treadmill exercise time of three minutes at one year. However, 31% of angioplasty patients and 22% of bypass graft patients still complained of anginal symptoms at two years. There was a marked difference in the rate of further revascularisation procedures, with 38% of the angioplasty group but only 11% of the bypass graft group having a further revascularisation procedure (or death or non-fatal infarction) within two years of randomisation. This study confirmed that both interventions were effective in relieving symptoms, and indistinguishable in terms of mortality or infarction outcomes, but patients randomised to angioplasty were much more likely to require a further revascularisation procedure, either in the form of further angioplasty or bypass grafting.

An important but poorly described use of angioplasty is in patients without overt effort-induced angina but with frequent hospital admissions on account of chest pain and one or more coronary artery stenoses on angiography.

Approximately 80% of coronary angioplasties in the United Kingdom are performed in patients with single-vessel coronary disease in whom long-term survival on medical therapy would be expected to be very good.[13]

Conclusions

Coronary bypass grafting and coronary angioplasty have been shown to improve survival in symptomatic patients with severe coronary artery disease. Both are also effective in relieving symptoms and in allowing the withdrawal of cardiac medication. Long-term results are probably better with coronary bypass grafting but at the price of increased early (perioperative) morbidity. In practice, because of limited availability of coronary bypass grafting, National Health Service patients in the UK are seldom offered a direct choice between bypass grafting and angioplasty; the former is offered if the patient falls into a group in which there is evidence of a survival benefit with surgery, the latter if the lesion is anatomically suitable and the procedure is being offered for the relief of symptoms rather than to improve survival. There is enormous variation in both bypass surgery and angioplasty rates between health regions in the UK, and between districts within regions. Even in the better resourced health care system in the USA, there are striking geographical practice variations. This may reflect different concepts of 'unacceptable symptoms' and different concepts of the extent to which management should be influenced by patient choice or by economic exigencies. Despite the potential risks, there is an impression that younger patients in particular would much prefer a 'one off' procedure to long-term medication.

References

1. Loop FD, Lytle BW, Cosgrove DM *et al.* Influence of the internal mammary artery graft on 10 year survival and other cardiac events. *New England Journal of Medicine* 1986; **314**: 1–6.
2. van der Meer J, Hillege HL, Kootstra GJ, Ascoop CAPL, Pfisterer M, van Gilst WH, Lie KI (for the CABADAS research group of the Interuniversity Cardiology Institute of the Netherlands). Prevention

of one year vein graft occlusion after aortocoronary bypass surgery: a comparison of low dose aspirin plus dipyridamole and oral anticoagulants. *Lancet* 1993; **342**: 257–63.

3. Gershlick AH, de Bono DP. Restenosis after angioplasty. *British Heart Journal* 1990; **64**: 351–3.

4. Varnauskas E and the European Coronary Surgery Study Group. Twelve year follow up of survival in the randomized European Coronary Surgery Study. *New England Journal of Medicine* 1988; **319**: 332–7.

5. Myers WO, Gersh BJ, Fisher L *et al.* Medical versus early surgical therapy in patients with triple vessel disease and mild angina pectoris: a CASS registry study of survival. *Annals of Thoracic Surgery* 1987; **44**: 471–86.

6. Myers WO, Schaff HV, Gersh BJ *et al.* Improved survival of surgically treated patients with triple vessel coronary artery disease and severe angina pectoris. A report from the Coronary Artery Surgery Study (CASS) registry. *Journal of Thoracic and Cardiovascular Surgery* 1989; **97**: 487–95.

7. Rogers WJ, Coggin CJ, Gersh BJ *et al.* Ten year follow up of quality of life in patients randomised to medicine vs. coronary artery bypass graft surgery, CASS. *Circulation* 1990; **82**: 1642–58.

8. Booth DC, Hultgren HN, Scott S, Luchi R, Dupree RH *et al.* Quality of life after bypass surgery for unstable angina: 5 year follow up results of a Veterans Administration Cooperative Study. *Circulation* 1991; **83**: 87–95.

9. Harrison MJG, Schniedau A, Ho R, Smith PLC, Treasure T. Cerebrovascular disease and functional outcome after coronary artery bypass surgery. *Stroke* 1989; **20**: 235–7.

10. Kirklin JW, Akins CW, Blackstone EH *et al.* Guidelines and indications for coronary artery bypass graft surgery. *Journal of the American College of Cardiology* 1991; **17**: 543–89.

11. Parisi AF, Folland ED, Hartigan P. A comparison of angioplasty with medical therapy in the treatment of single vessel coronary artery disease. *New England Journal of Medicine* 1992; **326**: 10–6.

12. RITA trial participants. Coronary angioplasty versus coronary artery bypass surgery: the randomised intervention treatment of angina (RITA) trial. *Lancet* 1993; **541**: 573–80.

13. Hubner PJBH. Cardiac interventional procedures in the United Kingdom in 1989. *British Heart Journal* 1991; **66**: 469–71.

8 | What happens in a district general hospital in the United Kingdom

John Birkhead

Consultant Physician, Northampton General Hospital

The incidence of stable angina pectoris within the population of the United Kingdom (UK) is not known with any certainty. The difficulties inherent in any examination of the incidence and prevalence of the condition have been examined in Chapters 2 and 3. The service provided to patients with angina pectoris is demand-led. Whilst increasing demand has been fuelled by increasing patient awareness and expectations, and particularly the reasonable expectations of older age groups,[1] the staffing and facilities that exist in some district hospitals in the UK may not be adequate to cope with these demands.

A large proportion of patients presenting in the community with angina pectoris will be referred initially by their general practitioner to a district general hospital; only a minority, usually for geographical reasons, will be referred directly to cardiac centres. The NHS and Community Care Act 1990 has not yet had any noticeable impact on local referral patterns, although this may change with the increase in the numbers of fundholding general practices.

Medical staffing

The manner in which angina pectoris is managed in a district general hospital depends on the medical and paramedical staffing available in relation to the workload.

Consultant staffing

Working in most district hospitals there will be a cardiologist who will have received formal training in the specialty, including training in invasive procedures. He or she will be fully accredited in cardiology and probably in general medicine as well. Cardiological physicians who have been appointed recently will often have their own catheter sessions at a local regional cardiac centre and will be able to study their own patients with ischaemic heart disease. Such an

71

arrangement is attractive, and allows vital contact with other cardiologists on a regular basis. There may not, however, be time to do this,
and to provide all the other essential services required of a cardiologist within the district hospital. The number of large district general hospitals in the UK (catchment population more than 250,000)
that have two cardiologists is small,[2,3] yet it is in these hospitals that
the investigative workload is greatest, and the time available for the
cardiologist to do his own invasive procedures will be shortest.

Whilst most district general hospitals have a cardiologist, there
remain more than 30 out of 215 district general hospitals, not
all small, where there is no trained cardiologist, or even a physician
devoting more than 40% of his or her time to the specialty.[2] In
these hospitals one of several physicians might deal with patients
with angina as outpatient referrals, and each physician may have a
different management policy. Some policies may not be appropriate in the light of present knowledge, and will be reflected in different thresholds for investigation and referral. Even in those hospitals with a cardiologist, elderly patients may not come under the
care of the cardiologist and may be managed differently.[1]

When considering the workload of a cardiologist, the numbers
of other consultant staff within the department of medicine is also
relevant. In smaller districts, with four or less physicians in general
medicine, the cardiovascular physician will have to shoulder more
of the general medical workload and even develop an interest in
another specialty in order to maintain services across the medical
spectrum.

Junior staff

At present, cardiovascular physicians in district general hospitals are
unlikely to have junior staff who are specifically training in cardiology. With the development of career registrar rotations with regional
cardiac centres, this is likely to change for a proportion of cardiovascular physicians, but it is unlikely, given the numbers in training in
the specialty, that more than a minority of district hospital cardiologists will be helping to train staff with some earlier formal training
in the specialty. Most will have a rotating registrar, or a senior house
officer, perhaps on a general practice vocational training scheme—a
young doctor with no long-term interest in cardiology.

Paramedical staff

There are difficulties in appointing, training and retaining

cardiovascular technicians in district hospitals.[4] Retaining trained
staff on uncompetitive salaries is particularly difficult in the South
of England. The lack of trained paramedical staff prevents appropriate use of facilities and results in medical staff performing
duties that could be performed by others.

Clinical audit

Single-handed consultants in any specialty will lack a yardstick with
which to compare the work of their department. Cardiologists are
heavy users of resources, both locally and in their referrals to cardiac centres; it is important for a cardiologist to know that his or
her referral patterns and other uses of resources are appropriate,
and that they should ensure that they liaise with other cardiological colleagues in their region for academic and audit purposes.

Source of patients

Although outpatient referrals might be expected to provide the
majority of patients with ischaemic heart disease, most patients
with angina come from among those discharged from the cardiac
care unit following an episode of acute coronary ischaemia, or
infarction. The annual figures from Northampton General Hospital illustrate this point. In the past three years, an average of 630
(range 600–680) new referrals have been seen for general practitioners. Slightly less than 25% are patients referred with chest
pain, of whom most have ischaemic heart disease. Thus about 130
(range 120–135) patients referred by their general practitioners
each year have ischaemic heart disease. By contrast, more than 500
patients are referred annually to the post-infarction clinic (400
patients/year aged 65 or under) following an admission to the
coronary care unit. In terms of subsequent referrals for angiography to the regional cardiac centre, about 50% of referrals have had
a recent infarction or episode of unstable angina, 25% have had an
infarct in the distant past, and a further 25% have angina without a
previous infarction. These proportions exclude those patients
referred directly as inpatients with unstable angina.

Outpatient management of patients referred with chest pain

It was stressed in *Achieving a Balance* stressed the need that more
patients should be seen by trained medical staff.[5] This is especially
important in outpatient clinics where a larger number of patients

are in contact with the hospital each year than are inpatients. An ideal clinic ratio of one consultant to one doctor in training is a rarity in a district hospital, and probably impracticable given the present staffing constraints within the UK. A larger number of consultants would allow certain benefits:

- More patients would be seen by trained staff
- Teaching of junior staff would improve
- Ratio of old to new patients would fall as a result of a more informed discharge policy.

Referral guidelines

Consultants and local general practitioners should agree guidelines for the management of angina for appropriate referral to the clinic. These should relate to national guidelines published after a critical appraisal of the scientific literature. They may prevent inappropriate referral and delay, and also remind practitioners of appropriate policies for investigation and the importance of lifestyle counselling. General practitioners and hospital staff should be clear about the local arrangements for seeing patients urgently, such as those presenting with rapidly progressive angina.

Post-infarction clinics

A trained cardiologist should see all patients following any episode of coronary ischaemia, in order that informed and consistent management should prevail in a group of patients who have a high incidence of serious pathology. In order to see 500 new patients annually (a typical figure for a catchment population of 250,000–300,000), and perhaps twice as many for review annually, the district cardiologist should set down clear written guidelines for junior staff, who change frequently, in order to provide a consistent service. The quality and commitment of junior staff vary, and the clinic will be seen by some juniors as a chore. It should be recognised that time for teaching in a clinic of this size will not be as much as is desirable. As any consultant will be on leave for approximately 12% of the year, the clinic, staffed purely by junior doctors during the absence of the consultant cardiologist, is likely to be of limited value during these periods. The need for two cardiologists in any district of more than 250,000 is only too apparent.[3]

Post-infarction clinics are valuable in the following ways:

- *Confirmation of the diagnosis and of the patient's understanding of the diagnosis.* Sometimes the patient has been misinformed of the correct diagnosis at some stage during the admission; more frequently, the patient has misunderstood what had been apparently clearly explained.

- *Assessment of progress since discharge.* Given the current financial pressures to discharge patients early, some patients will be discharged before a proper evaluation of left ventricular function. The diagnosis of minor degrees of left ventricular dysfunction in immobile patients is not easy, and heart failure is often only manifest on full mobilisation after the patient reaches home.
- *Review of therapy.* The clinic is a useful point at which to rationalise therapy. Beta-adrenergic blockers and enzyme converting inhibitors can usefully be introduced at this stage where appropriate.
- *Investigations.* Post-infarction exercise testing is usually performed at about one month after infarction; attendance at the post-infarction clinic is an appropriate moment to evaluate results. Echocardiographic assessment of ventricular function and 24-hour ambulatory monitoring can be performed as indicated.
- *Arrangements for coronary rehabilitation can be reviewed.*

Investigation of patients with suspected angina pectoris

Chest pain makes patients anxious, and often referral to hospital is necessary for reassurance rather than to exclude significant pathology. A carefully taken history will sort out many without further investigation. However, there are important differential diagnoses which require careful assessment and investigation. The more important that may cause diagnostic difficulty include hypertrophic cardiomyopathy (particularly in those presenting without obstructive features), hyperventilation syndrome, syndrome X, disorders of oesophageal motility, and oesophagitis. In each condition, symptoms indistinguishable from obstructive coronary artery disease can occur.

Exercise electrocardiography remains the main investigation performed in the evaluation of presumed angina pectoris within a district general hospital; it is discussed at length in Chapter 5. The use of ambulatory monitoring to assess silent ischaemia and the adjunctive use of nuclear studies to provide functional information are discussed below.

Nuclear cardiology

Radioisotope studies provide valuable functional information which is complementary to the anatomical information provided by angiography (Chapter 9). Despite this, radioisotope studies appear to play a limited part in the investigation of patients with coronary disease in a district general hospital in the UK. In the UK, cardiac studies represent only 11% of the total nuclear workload, and in district hospitals this figure is 7%.[6] The total number of cardiac studies performed in the UK approximates to 700/million/year compared with 4,000/million/year in the USA. Only about 50% (110/215) of district general hospitals use cardiac scintigraphy. There is a wide inter-regional variation; in the Mersey region, one of ten health districts uses scintigraphy whilst in the West Midlands region the figure is 15 of 22.

There are a number of possible reasons why the use of radioisotope techniques is not more widespread. There are financial constraints which limit the use of nuclear studies within district hospitals, and not least the constraints of time upon the single-handed cardiologist. There is also a lack of formal training in nuclear cardiology for cardiologists and radiologists in training; radiologists often do not perform the procedures, but they frequently report them. Patients in whom nuclear investigations appear to be most valuable are those with the greatest diagnostic uncertainty, such as equivocal or uninterpretable exercise tests; these represent the minority of those tested. If nuclear investigation is limited to those in whom there is genuine diagnostic difficulty, the number of investigations performed will be limited. As expertise only comes with constant practice, the numbers performed in a district hospital may be too small for the cardiologist or reporting radiologist to maintain diagnostic competence. As nuclear studies are most valuable in complementing the angiographic findings, they are more appropriately performed at the same time and place as angiography.

Evaluation of silent ischaemia

Studies have shown that asymptomatic ischaemia demonstrated on ambulatory monitoring provides additional independent prognostic information.[7] Pain thresholds vary,[8] especially in the elderly,[9] and possibly also in diabetics. No figures are available for the frequency with which ambulatory monitoring of silent ischaemia is performed in district hospitals; constraints of time, equipment, and a lack of conviction about the value of the additional information provided by the technique may all be relevant.

Selection of patients with established coronary disease for angiography

This difficult topic is more fully discussed in Chapter 7, but I stress the following points. A number of studies have shown that the prognosis of a proportion of patients with symptomatically mild coronary disease is better after surgical than medical treatment.[10-12] It follows that all patients with angina should have angiography, and this is manifestly not the case in the UK. The factors that influence the decision to refer a patient for angiography are:

- Severity of symptoms in relation to age, and to the expectations/needs of the patient
- Co-existent disease
- Length of history, a longer history being associated with a poorer prognosis
- Previous infarction
- Response to, and tolerability of, drug therapy
- Response to exercise testing:
  Early symptoms: <6 min Bruce protocol or equivalent
  Poor haemodynamic response/maximum workload
  Prolonged ST segment depression
  Early/deep ST depression (with or without symptoms)
  Ventricular arrhythmias

The ability of the regional cardiac centre to accept work may be an (unconscious) determinant of threshold for referral, and the knowledge that angiography may be followed by a prolonged further wait for surgery may influence its timing.

The future

The place of angiography within hospitals without on-site access to cardiac surgery has been controversial, but district hospital cardiologists are now performing on-site coronary angiography more frequently. Further expansion of angiography in district general hospitals seems likely to happen for a number of reasons. The demand for angiography is increasing, and experience suggests that this demand already appears to be beyond the ability of regional cardiac centres to cope. As more younger cardiologists are appointed to district hospitals, the demand for many of them to have investigative facilities in regional centres will exceed the available facilities; these cardiologists will wish to develop angiography facilities within their own district. The cost of setting up cardiac angiography facilities is well within the reach of any district hospital that already has a general angiography suite within the radiology department. More intensive use of expensive radiological equipment not fully utilised in general angiography is an additional advantage. There are advantages to coronary angiography within a district hospital, which include a greater potential for day case procedures than is the case at a regional centre, and better access for patients. Great care will have to be exercised in determining suitable patients for on-site angiography; high risk patients will need to be studied at the regional cardiac centre. If coronary angiography becomes widespread in district hospitals, stringent quality assurance will become a prerequisite.

The rate of expansion in the specialty is slow.[2] Given the current constraints upon consultant expansion, which may be exacerbated by the new contracting arrangements, and the limited number of senior registrars in training, it is unlikely that a useful increase in the numbers of cardiologists will occur. Short-term expediency has dictated the appointment of staff grade physicians to cover the workload in some districts. Such appointments should not be permitted to inhibit or suppress the need for consultant expansion. It is, unfortunately, relatively easy to appoint to a staff grade post compared with the difficulties of funding and appointing a new consultant cardiologist.

Conclusion

Improvements in the management of angina pectoris in district hospitals will only come about with improved staffing, both with fully trained cardiologists and appropriate paramedical support. A reduction in mortality from coronary disease is one of the targets of *The Health of the Nation.*[13] This will not be achieved without appropriate investment in staff and equipment. The majority of ischaemic heart disease presents initially to district hospitals; it is logical that much of the investment must be made there.

Acknowledgments

The author thanks Dr Jane Flint for help with drafting the section on nuclear cardiology.

References

1. Royal College of Physicians of London. Cardiological interventions for elderly patients: report of joint working group, 1991.

2. Chamberlain D, Pentecost B, Reval *et al.* Staffing in cardiology in the United Kingdom 1990. Sixth biennial survey: with data on facilities in cardiology in England and Wales. *British Heart Journal* 1991; **66**: 395–404.

3. Royal College of Surgeons and Royal College of Physicians. Provision of services for the diagnosis and treatment of heart disease: fourth report of joint cardiology committee. 1991. *British Heart Journal* 1992; **67**: 106–16.

4. British Cardiac Society. Cardiology in the district hospital: report of a working group. *British Heart Journal* 1987; **58**: 537–46.

5. *Achieving a balance.* London: HMSO, 1987; Section B: para 6.

6. Underwood R, Gibson C, Tweddel A, Flint J, on behalf of the British Nuclear Cardiology Group. A survey of nuclear cardiological practice in Great Britain. *British Heart Journal* 1992; **67**: 273–7.

7. Deedwania P, Carbajal E. Silent ischaemia during daily life is an independent predictor of mortality in stable angina. *Circulation* 1990; **81**: 748–56.

8. Glazier J, Chierchia S, Brown M, Maseri A. Importance of generalised defective perception of painful stimuli as a cause of silent myocardial ischaemia in chronic stable angina pectoris. *American Journal of Cardiology* 1986; **58**: 667–72.

9. Miller P, Sheps D, Bragdon E *et al.* Ageing and pain perception in ischaemic heart disease. *American Heart Journal* 1990; **120**: 22–30.

10. CASS investigators. Coronary artery surgery study (CASS): a randomised trial of coronary artery bypass surgery: survival data. *Circulation* 1983; **68**: 939–50.

11. European Coronary Surgery Study Group. Long term results of prospective randomised study of coronary artery bypass surgery in stable angina patients. *Lancet* 1982; **ii**: 1173–80.

12. Survival of patients with mild angina or myocardial infarction without angina: a comparison of medical and surgical treatment. *British Heart Journal* 1988; **59**: 641–7.

13. Department of Health. *The Health of the Nation.* London: HMSO, 1992.

9 | Role of myocardial perfusion imaging in coronary artery disease

Dudley Pennell and Richard Underwood

Senior Lecturers in Cardiac Imaging, Royal Brompton National Heart and Lung Hospital, London

Whilst typical angina is a good indicator of myocardial ischaemia, and abolition of symptoms is an important aim of treatment, stable symptoms indicate neither the site or extent of ischaemia nor the likely risk of future cardiac events. In many cases, it is helpful to have an objective assessment of myocardial ischaemia in order to guide future management, and myocardial perfusion scintigraphy is the only non-invasive and widely available method of assessing myocardial perfusion. It therefore has an obvious role in the detection of perfusion abnormalities caused by coronary artery disease.

Diagnosis of coronary artery disease

Many studies have assessed the sensitivity and specificity of myocardial perfusion imaging for the detection of coronary artery disease, the coronary arteriogram usually being used as the standard by which the accuracy of scintigraphy is judged. The wisdom of this approach can be debated, but at least the arteriogram provides a universal standard for coronary arterial anatomy even if it is a less good standard by which to judge coronary arterial function. A review of 15 studies, involving 1,501 patients,[1] found an overall sensitivity and specificity for the detection of coronary artery disease of 80% and 92%, which was significantly better than with exercise electrocardiography (64% and 82% respectively). Comparisons using receiver operating curve analysis, which tests one technique against another over a range of possible diagnostic thresholds, have also confirmed the superior diagnostic capabilities of perfusion imaging.[2]

It is reasonable to ask therefore whether thallium scintigraphy should be used in place of exercise electrocardiography for the diagnosis of suspected coronary artery disease. Several factors militate against this, particularly in the UK, where the lower availability of thallium imaging, poor training in the use of the technique, and inexperienced interpreters will also influence the decision. Additional important factors are the radiation burden to the patient and the additional expense. Therefore, for the *diagnosis* of coronary artery disease, thallium imaging is usefully employed where exercise electrocardiography is unhelpful or leaves doubt. In clinical practice this may occur when: resting ECG changes are present (left bundle branch block, pre-excitation, left ventricular hypertrophy, drug effects etc), equivocal ST segment changes occur with exercise, a normal exercise electrocardiogram occurs despite a high pre-test likelihood of disease, abnormal ST segment changes are seen despite a low pre-test likelihood of disease, or only submaximal exercise is achieved (pharmacological thallium imaging is ideal in these patients). However, it must always be borne in mind that the diagnostic capabilities of any investigation depend on the likelihood of disease in the population under test, and thallium imaging is subject to these constraints.

The concept of pre-test and post-test likelihood of disease arises from Bayes' theorem which is central to the correct application of any diagnostic test.[3,4] The theorem predicts that the greatest contribution to diagnosis from a test that is similar in sensitivity and specificity to thallium scintigraphy is made when the pre-test likelihood of disease is around 50%. When the pre-test likelihood of disease is very low, even an abnormal test does not increase the likelihood of disease by very much. Conversely, a normal test in a patient with a very high pre-test likelihood does not significantly lower the likelihood of disease. It is always worth considering the pre-test likelihood of disease before requesting a diagnostic test with less than perfect sensitivity and specificity.

Prognosis and coronary artery disease

The most valuable contribution that nuclear techniques can make to the management of patients with coronary artery disease is to assess the future risk of myocardial infarction and death. Prognosis has long been known to depend upon the severity of the coronary disease but the problem lies in an objective assessment of *severity*. Coronary arteriography is commonly used to assess the number of diseased vessels and the site of the lesions; however, this is a crude method of assessing the functional significance of disease. Visual assessment of coronary arteriograms has long been known to have a large intraobserver and interobserver variability[5,6] and a poor association with post mortem anatomy.[7-9] More recently, poor relationship between luminal narrowing and coronary function has also been demonstrated.[10] Some attempt can be made to improve the assessment using either a coronary artery score[11-13] or digitised tracing of the lesions to combine the effects of luminal narrowing and length and morphology of the stenosis.[14] This is complicated by the fact that coronary arteries are not passive conduits but active organs[15] that control the shear stress along their walls by dilating in response to increases in flow.[16] This normal dilation is impaired or reversed by atheromatous disease.[17] There can be no doubt therefore that coronary artery function must be assessed by a separate technique and that the main role of coronary arteriography is as an anatomical guide for angioplasty or surgery.

Exercise electrocardiography is the most commonly performed of the tests of coronary function. Several parameters can provide prognostic information including exercise time, ST segment depression and blood pressure response,[18-20] but all of these are relatively crude measures of the extent of ischaemia. Exercise radionuclide ventriculography provides a more refined assessment because abnormal regional contraction is an early manifestation of reversible ischaemia. Extensive abnormalities impair left ventricular ejection fraction which is an excellent indicator of prognosis.[21-23] Measurements made during exercise are superior to measurements at rest because they reflect the extent of infarction and of reversible ischaemia.

Because it is the extent of jeopardised myocardium that determines risk, it is most rational to look at myocardial perfusion directly. The evidence that thallium myocardial perfusion imaging provides important prognostic information in stable angina,[24-26] and following myocardial infarction,[27,28] is overwhelming.[29] This information is present in the scan irrespective of the stress used, and assessment of problem patients by pharmacological stress may be valuable.[30-32] Both the extent and the severity of reversible defects are independent predictors of cardiac events at one year,[33] with the cardiac event rate varying from 0.4% in patients with normal exercise perfusion to 78% in patients with both severe and extensive perfusion defects. Myocardial perfusion imaging is superior to exercise electrocardiography for defining prognosis.[34] Comparisons of thallium imaging with coronary angiography have also shown thallium imaging to have greater and incremental[35,36] prognostic power.[24,26,27] It is also important to note the significance of a normal thallium scan, because the event rate in these patients is low, being less than 1%. Many patients with atypical chest pain can be strongly reassured on this basis,[37-39] and the low risk appears to last for up to 10 years.[40] The final use of the prognostic power of thallium imaging is in assessing cardiac risk associated with non-cardiac surgery. This is particularly important for patients with limited exercise capabilities, such as those undergoing peripheral vascular reconstruction, because pharmacological stress may be performed.[41-43] Results show that patients with reversible ischaemia are at greater risk than those with normal scans or with fixed defects only, and that the thallium assessment is superior to both clinical variables and the exercise electrocardiogram.[44-46]

Thus it could be argued that myocardial perfusion imaging should be performed in all patients with coronary artery disease in order to assess prognosis and to select patients who, irrespective of symptoms, deserve angiography with a view to intervention in order to prevent future infarction or death. However, if myocardial perfusion imaging is the most effective way of assessing prognosis in patients with coronary artery disease, the question of whether it should be used to assess patients who have minimal or no symptoms will depend on whether the prognosis in such patients is further improved by interventions directed at correcting large areas of reversible ischaemia. Direct evidence on this point is not yet available, but the poor correlation between symptoms and prognosis suggests that a decision to intervene based on severely adverse prognostic indicators should not be prevented by the symptomatic status.

The powerful prognostic value of myocardial perfusion imaging is difficult to square with the increasing evidence that the degree to which coronary atheroma impairs coronary flow reserve is not necessarily related to the instability of the lesion and hence the risk of coronary thrombosis. Only one third of infarctions occur because of occlusion of the most severe stenosis, and two thirds occur at stenoses that were less than 50%.[47-49] Thus there will always be patients who present with myocardial infarction or sudden death without preceding angina, and we do not yet have a diagnostic technique that is capable of detecting such early lesions. Presumably the prognostic power of myocardial perfusion imaging arises from the fact that patients with extensive flow-limiting lesions are also likely to have thrombogenic lesions (even if not flow-limiting) and so are at high risk of infarction.

References

1. Rozanski A, Berman DS. The efficacy of cardiovascular nuclear medicine exercise studies. *Seminars in Nuclear Medicine* 1987; **17**:104–20.

2. Morise AP, Detrano R, Bobbio M, Diamond GA. Development and validation of a logistic regression-derived algorithm for estimating the incremental probability of coronary artery disease before and after exercise testing. *Journal of the American College of Cardiology* 1992; **20:**1187–96.

3. Diamond GA. Reverend Bayes' silent majority. An alternative factor affecting sensitivity and specificity of exercise electrocardiography. *American Journal of Cardiology* 1986; **57:** 1175–9.

4. Detrano R, Leatherman J, Salcedo EE, Yiannikas J, Williams G. Bayesian analysis versus discriminant function analysis: their relative utility in the diagnosis of coronary disease. *Circulation* 1986;**73:** 970–7.

5. Zir LM, Miller SW, Dinsmore RH, Gilbert JP, Harthorne JW. Inter-observer variability in coronary angiography. *Circulation* 1976; **53:** 627–32.

6. Galbraith JE, Murphy L, Desoyza N. Coronary angiogram interpretation: interobserver variability. *Journal of the American Medical Association* 1981; **240:** 2053–6.

7. Grodin CM, Dyrda I, Pasternac A, Campeau L, Bourassa MG. Discrepancies between cine angiographic and post-mortem findings in patients with coronary artery disease and recent myocardial revascularisation. *Circulation* 1974; **49:** 703–8.

8. Isner JM, Kishel J, Kent KM. Accuracy of angiographic determination of left main coronary arterial narrowing. *Circulation* 1981; **63:** 1056–64.

9. Roberts WC, Jones AA. Quantitation of coronary arterial narrowing at necropsy in sudden coronary death. *American Journal of Cardiology* 1979; **44:** 39–45.

10. White CW, Wright CB, Doty DB, *et al.* Does visual interpretation of the coronary arteriogram predict the physiologic importance of a coronary stenosis? *New England Journal of Medicine* 1984;**310:** 819–24.

11. Balcon R. Prognostic significance of coronary angiography. *European Heart Journal* 1984; **5:** 73–5.

12. Balcon R. The relationship between prognosis and angiographic and exercise data. *Acta Medica Scandinavica* 1984; **694 (suppl):** 101–3.

13. Moise A, Clement B, Saltiel J. Clinical and angiographic correlates and prognostic significance of the coronary extent score. *American Journal of Cardiology* 1988; **61:** 1255–9.

14. Nissen SE, Gurley JC. Assessment of the functional significance of coronary stenoses. Is digital angiography the answer? *Circulation* 1990; **81:** 1431–5.

15. Chesebro JH, Fuster V, Webster MWI. Editorial comment. Endothelial injury and coronary vasomotion. *Journal of the American College of Cardiology* 1989; **14:** 1191–2.

16. Bing RJ. Editorial comment. Control of shear stress in the epicardial coronary arteries of humans: impairment by atherosclerosis. *Journal of the American College of Cardiology* 1989; **14:** 1200–1.

17. Vita JA, Treasure CB, Ganz P, Cox DA, Fish RD, Selwyn AP. Control of shear stress in the epicardial coronary arteries of humans: impairment by atherosclerosis. *Journal of the American College of Cardiology* 1989; **14:** 1193–9.

18. Rautaharju PM, Prineas RJ, Eifler WJ, *et al.* Prognostic value of exercise electrocardiogram in men at high risk of future coronary heart disease: multiple risk factor intervention trial experience. *Journal of the American College of Cardiology* 1986: **8:** 1–10.

19. Stone PH, Turi ZG, Muller JE, *et al.* Prognostic significance of the treadmill exercise test performance 6 months after myocardial infarction. *Journal of the American College of Cardiology* 1986; **8:** 1007–17.

20. Goldschlager N, Sox HC. The diagnostic and prognostic value of the treadmill exercise test in the evaluation of chest pain, in patients with recent myocardial infarction and in asymptomatic individuals. *American Heart Journal* 1988; **116:** 523–35.

21. Bonow RO, Kent KM, Rosing DR, *et al.* Exercise-induced ischaemia in mildly symptomatic patients with coronary artery disease, and preserved left ventricular function: identification of subgroups at high risk for death during medical therapy. *New England Journal of Medicine* 1984; **311:** 1339–45.

22. Iskandrian AS, Hakki AH, Goel IP, Mundth ED, Kane-Marsch SA, Schenk CL. Use of rest and exercise radionuclide ventriculography in risk stratification in patients with suspected coronary artery disease. *American Heart Journal* 1985; **110:** 864–72.

23. Abraham RD, Harris PJ, Roubin GS, *et al.* Usefulness of ejection fraction response to exercise one month after acute myocardial infarction in predicting coronary anatomy and prognosis. *American Journal of Cardiology* 1987; **60:** 225–30.

24. Brown KA, Boucher CA, Okada RD, *et al.* Prognostic value of exercise thallium-201 imaging in patients presenting for evaluation of chest pain. *Journal of the American College of Cardiology* 1983; **1:** 994–1001.

25. Iskandrian AS, Heo J, Decoskey D, Askenase A, Segal BL. Use of exercise thallium-201 imaging for risk stratification of elderly patients with coronary artery disease. *American Journal of Cardiology* 1988; **61:** 269–72.

26. Kaul S, Finkelstein DM, Homma S, Leavitt M, Okada RD, Boucher CA. Superiority of quantitative exercise thallium-201 variables in determining long-term prognosis in ambulatory patients with chest pain: a comparison with cardiac catheterization. *Journal of the American College of Cardiology* 1988; **12:** 25–34.

27. Gibson RS, Watson DD, Craddock GB, *et al.* Prediction of cardiac events after uncomplicated myocardial infarction: a prospective study comparing predischarge exercise thallium-201 scintigraphy and coronary angiography. *Circulation* 1983; **68:** 321–6.

28. Wilson WW, Gibson RS, Nygaard TW, *et al.* Acute myocardial infarction associated with single vessel coronary artery disease: an analysis of clinical outcome and the prognostic importance of vessel patency and residual ischemic myocardium. *Journal of the American College of Cardiology* 1988; **11:** 223–34.

29. Brown KA. Prognostic value of thallium-201 myocardial perfusion imaging. A diagnostic tool comes of age. *Circulation* 1991; **83:** 363–81.

30. Gimple DW, Hutter AM, Guiney TE, Boucher CA. Prognostic utility of predischarge dipyridamole-thallium imaging compared to predischarge submaximal exercise electrocardiography and maximal

exercise thallium imaging after uncomplicated acute myocardial infarction. *American Journal of Cardiology* 1989; **64**: 1243–8.

31. Younis LT, Byers S, Shaw L, Barth G, Goodgold H, Chaitman BR. Prognostic value of intravenous dipyridamole thallium scintigraphy after an acute myocardial ischemic event. *American Journal of Cardiology* 1989; **64:** 161–6.

32. Leppo JA, O'Brien J, Rothendler JA, Getchèll JD, Lee VW. Dipyridamole-thallium-201 scintigraphy in the prediction of future cardiac events after acute myocardial infarction. *New England Journal of Medicine* 1984; **310:** 1014–8.

33. Ladenheim ML, Pollock BH, Rozanski A, *et al.* Extent and severity of myocardial perfusion as predictors of prognosis in patients with suspected coronary artery disease. *Journal of the American College of Cardiology* 1986; **7:** 464–71.

34. Ladenheim ML, Kotler TS, Pollock BH, Berman DS, Diamond DA. Incremental prognostic power of clinical history, exercise electrocardiography and myocardial perfusion scintigraphy in suspected coronary artery disease. *American Journal of Cardiology* 1987; **59:** 270–7.

35. Iskandrian AS, Chae SC, Heo J, Stanberry CD, Wasserleben V, Cave V. Independent and incremental prognostic value of exercise single photon emission computed tomography (SPECT) thallium imaging in coronary artery disease. *Journal of the American College of Cardiology* 1993; **22:** 665–70.

36. Kaul S, Lilly DR, Gascho JA, *et al.* Prognostic utility of the exercise thallium-201 test in ambulatory patients with chest pain: comparison with cardiac catheterisation. *Circulation* 1988; **77:** 745–58.

37. Wackers EJ, Russo DS, Russo D, Clements JP. Prognostic significance of normal quantitative planar thallium-201 stress scintigraphy in patients with chest pain. *Journal of the American College of Cardiology* 1985; **6:** 27–32.

38. Oosterhuis WP, Breeman A, Niemeyer MG, *et al.* Patients with a normal exercise thallium-201 myocardial scintigram—always a good prognosis. *European Journal of Nuclear Medicine* 1993; **20:** 151–8.

39. Brown KA, Rowen M. Prognostic value of a normal exercise myocardial perfusion imaging study in patients with angiographically significant coronary artery disease. *American Journal of Cardiology* 1993; **71:** 865–7.

40. Steinberg EH, Koss JH, Lee M, Grunwald AM, Bodenheimer MM. Prognostic significance from 10 year follow up of a qualitatively normal planar exercise thallium test in suspected coronary artery disease. *American Journal of Cardiology* 1993; **71:** 1270–3.

41. Fletcher JP, Antico VF, Gruenewald S, Kershaw LZ. Dipyridamole-thallium scan for screening of coronary artery disease prior to vascular surgery. *Journal of Cardiovascular Surgery* 1988; **29:** 666–9.

42. Lette J, Waters D, Lapointe J, *et al.* Usefulness of the severity and extent of reversible perfusion defects during thallium-dipyridamole imaging for cardiac risk assessment before noncardiac surgery. *American Journal of Cardiology* 1989; **64:** 276–81.

43. Sachs RN, Tellier P, Larmignat P, *et al.* Assessment by dipyridamole thallium-201 myocardial scintigraphy of coronary risk before peripheral vascular surgery. *Surgery* 1988; **103:** 584–7.

44. Leppo J, Plaja J, Gionet M, Tumolo J, Paraskos JA, Cutler BS. Non-invasive evaluation of cardiac risk before elective vascular surgery. *Journal of the American College of Cardiology* 1987; **9:** 269–76.
45. Reifsnyder T, Randyk DF, Lanza D, Seabrook GR, Towne JB. Use of stress thallium imaging to stratify cardiac risk in patients undergoing vascular surgery. *Journal of Surgical Research* 1992; **52:** 147–51.
46. Coley CM, Field TS, Abraham SA, Boucher CA, Eagle KA. Usefulness of dipyridamole thallium scanning for pre-operative evaluation of cardiac risk for non-vascular surgery. *American Journal of Cardiology* 1992; **69:** 1280–5.
47. Little WC, Constantinescu M, Applegate RJ, *et al.* Can coronary angiography predict the site of a subsequent myocardial infarction in patients with mild-to-moderate coronary artery disease? *Circulation* 1988; **78:** 1157–66.
48. Hackett D, Davies G, Maseri A. Pre-existing coronary stenoses in patients with first myocardial infarction are not necessarily severe. *European Heart Journal* 1988; **9:** 1317–23.
49. Brosius FC, Roberts WC. Comparison of degree and extent of coronary narrowing by atherosclerotic plaque in anterior and posterior transmural acute myocardial infarction. *Circulation* 1981; **64:** 715–22.

10 | The district general hospital and its relationship to the specialist cardiac centre

Michael Joy
Consultant Physician and Cardiologist,
St Peter's Hospital, Chertsey, Surrey

There has been a substantial growth in the past two decades in both the pharmacological and the interventional techniques available to the cardiologist for the management of the various coronary syndromes. Thrombolytic agents, beta-blocking agents and angiotensin converting enzyme inhibitors have been shown to enhance survival overall following myocardial infarction, and angiotensin converting enzyme inhibitors are effective in prolonging survival of patients with impairment of ventricular function from whatever cause. However, none of these potential benefits is available without adequate specialist provision and diagnostic facilities, all of which should be available in a district hospital.

Development of a cardiological service in the United Kingdom

Ten years ago, Chamberlain *et al.* reviewed career prospects in cardiology in England and Wales.[1] There were then only 103 physicians fully committed to the specialty, with 98 further physicians spending more than 40% of their time in it. There were 22 paediatric cardiologists. This small number of specialists was attempting to provide care for a population of some 46 million people. Inevitably this was piecemeal, and a substantial proportion of the population lived in health districts that did not have a physician trained in cardiology on the staff of the local district general hospital.

At much the same time, the second report of the joint cardiology committee of the Royal College of Physicians of London and the Royal College of Surgeons of England made recommendations on the size, workload, siting and staffing of modern combined cardiological/cardiac surgical facilities.[2] Almost for the first time, attention was drawn to the need for hospitals without cardiac surgical facilities to provide for the care of cardiac emergencies. There was also a need for non-invasive investigative techniques including Holter monitoring, echocardiography and exercise electrocardiography. Close liaison between the subsidiary centre at the district general hospital and the specialist cardiac centre was recommended. Other initiatives such as the development of clinics for the management of hypertension and for cardiac rehabilitation were felt to be desirable.

A smaller proportion of gross domestic product is allocated to health care in the UK than in any country in Europe other than Greece,[3] and to some extent this has held back the growth of specialist medicine. Chamberlain and his colleagues, in a series of reviews of staffing, have repeatedly drawn attention to the shortcomings of staffing at consultant level in cardiology.[4-7] Even by 1990, 44 of 218 health districts in England and Wales with a population of 8.3 million people had no full-time physician trained in cardiology.[8] The limited availability of cardiologists has led to lower demand for specialist services than would be predicted from the known epidemiology of coronary disease and the known efficacy of available treatment. It has held back the substantial pressure for expansion, notably in investigative services as well as in the provision of cardiac surgery. National levels of activity in terms of cardiac catheterisation and cardiopulmonary bypass procedures do not give an accurate statement of need, as those health districts without a cardiologist have a significantly lower uptake of the facilities at specialist cardiac centres. Likewise the development of specialist care services in district hospitals is slower in the absence of a specialist. These difficulties were brought into focus by a working group of the British Cardiac Society which concerned itself exclusively with the problems of cardiology in the district hospital.[8]

Cardiological services in the district general hospital

Joy and Hugget[9] recorded the first experience of a district hospital cardiological unit set up along the lines suggested by the second joint report of the Royal Colleges.[2] They pointed out that the level of activity they experienced was to some extent related to their ability to provide services rather than to the need for them. Based on their experience, the authors made suggestions on staffing, including technical staff, and on the number of investigations that might be expected to be performed in a typical health district. This early report was followed by that of a working group of the British Cardiac Society.[8] This survey contained a summary of data

obtained from 65 responding hospitals out of a total of 172 originally approached about their facilities and their levels of activity.
Those who responded varied widely in terms of activity and
appeared to be increasing their workload steadily. The report recommended that every district hospital should have at least one
physician trained in cardiology (two if the catchment population
exceeded 250,000), that such a catchment population required a
department with seven technicians of appropriate grade mix, working in an area of not less than 3,000 square feet, and that all modern non-invasive investigative facilities should be available.[8] Each
unit should develop a close working relationship with a specialist
cardiac centre or centres. The British Cardiac Society has recently
commissioned a follow-up report. Recent developments following
the purchaser/provider split in the NHS are likely to lead to a
smaller number of larger district units.

Table 1. Estimated minimum need for non-invasive investigation compared with number of procedures carried out in a typical district hospital;
expressed per 100,000 population per year.[8]

Resting ECG	5,000	3,000
Exercise electrocardiograms	300	200
Echocardiograms	300	250
Ambulatory ECG	250	150

Provision of cardiological services by specialist cardiac centres

The specialist cardiac centre provides a full range of diagnostic
and interventional services for its own catchment population and
those services that are not available at district level. The district
health authority will contract for such specialist services. They
should, but commonly do not, involve the local cardiologist in
negotiations. Fundholding general practitioners may seek to
bypass their local centre, for whatever reason, and send their
patients directly to a specialist centre, which is likely to have higher
costs and therefore charges. The centre will also provide a reference point for the district hospital cardiologist, often working in
isolation, when additional expertise is required, such as in the
management of complex arrhythmias.
      On the grounds of cost, ease of patient access and immediacy of

care for those conditions that need urgent intervention, such as the acute coronary syndromes, it is appropriate that a patient be seen at least initially at district level. Any onward referral should be for specific services such as investigation, eg cardiac catheterisation, or treatment, eg surgery or percutaneous coronary angioplasty. The suggestion that the district cardiologist should be the budgetary gatekeeper for such activity is so obvious that it is unlikely to be adopted.

Need for further investigation and surgery

Specialist cardiac centres with a defined catchment population have been slow to analyse their service provision in a way that answers the question of what need there is for invasive investigation and revascularisation procedures in the United Kingdom. What has been published is often speculative.[10] However, some new data have recently become available.[11]

In order to define the population need for those procedures that cannot be provided by the district general hospital, the activity of the cardiological unit at St Peter's Hospital has been audited continuously since 1979 and has yielded increasingly useful information.[9,12,13] The data collected are based on a relatively static population after careful review of patient movement across the boundaries of the district health authority. North West Surrey health district (before the recent boundary change) had a standardised mortality ratio (SMR) approximately half that of Ayrshire; for coronary heart deaths the SMR at 0.78 is almost bottom of the national league. Corrections therefore have to be applied before our observations can be extrapolated to a regional or national requirement for invasive investigation and cardiopulmonary bypass procedures.

Different health districts have differing requirements of specialist cardiac centres, reflecting not only their local incidence of cardiac disease but also a diversity of other differences including geographical location (there is a north/south gradient in the prevalence of coronary artery disease), social deprivation (coronary artery disease is skewed towards lower socio-economic groups) and, increasingly, ethnic differences (there is a higher prevalence of coronary artery disease amongst patients from the Indian subcontinent). Taking these variations into account, the North West Surrey data suggest that there is a national need for between 700 and 1,000 coronary angiograms and 390 and 600 coronary artery bypass procedures per million population per annum.[13] The data were too few to permit an assessment of the need for percutaneous transluminal coronary angioplasty, but there appears to be a further requirement for 70 valvar heart operations (and associated cardiac catheterisation) and 30 other miscellaneous cardiac procedures per million population per annum. Early evidence from comparative trials of revascularisation by angioplasty or surgery, such as RITA,[14] do not lend support to the notion that angioplasty will reduce, even in part, the need for coronary artery surgery.

The rate of intervention on patients with valvar heart disease did not change over the ten-year period under review, while coronary artery surgery has shown an almost exponential increase. Unpublished data from our department suggest that this rate of increase has flattened off, and that the ongoing requirement of North West Surrey for coronary angiography and coronary artery bypass grafting is likely to remain at or about the level of 1988. However, this takes no account of the impact of coronary angioplasty although this may be smaller than anticipated.[14]

Relationship between a district hospital and a specialist centre

Professional relationships

A properly established district centre will normally expect to provide consultant services and non-invasive investigative facilities. Although occasionally a 'second opinion' may be sought of a colleague in a specialist centre, the great majority of referrals from the district hospital will be for invasive investigation and surgery as isolated items of service. Depending on individual arrangements, the district hospital cardiologist may visit the specialist centre regularly to perform investigation on his own patients. Not all do. Whatever the arrangement, it should be possible for patients to be placed directly on the waiting list at the specialist centre without the need for outpatient episodes which reduplicate effort and are costly and wasteful. Only those services not available at the district hospital should be provided for its patients at the specialist centre.

The issue as to responsibility for patient care is not completely straightforward. When making a referral to the specialist centre, a district cardiologist recognises that, as in his own hospital, the patient may be investigated by a doctor still in training. In the past, some patients have been investigated by visiting junior colleagues under training who are not part of an approved training programme, often by a research fellow attached to an academic department. Most district cardiologists (on behalf of their patients) would expect their patients to be investigated, if not by a consultant, by a senior registrar, or a regional registrar who is either competent or properly supervised. In future, purchasers may make this a contractual requirement.

The role of the district cardiologist. In North West Surrey, for many years, there has been an agreement that all referrals to the specialist centre should be through the district cardiologist.[9] Increasingly, general medicine has become specialised; the district cardiologist is in the best position to make judgments about the deployment of increasingly scarce resources in his or her specialty. Unfortunately, the issue of clinical freedom is sometimes raised to counter such an approach and, in certain districts in which there are well developed local cardiological facilities, physicians who are specialists in other disciplines insist on their right to refer directly to the specialist centre. Commissioners or purchasers of cardiac care may be best advised to permit the district cardiologist to act as surrogate budget holder in the disbursement of district funds for the purchase of services from the specialist centre.

Direct general practitioner referrals to the specialist cardiac centre. Specialist centres are likely to encourage direct referral from general practitioners when they are fundholders. Such direct referrals often have real disadvantages for the patients who are required to travel significant distances for services that can be provided close at hand and of which the patient may not be aware. The district unit is likely to have to provide acute services following any mishap, so it is helpful if information following such an episode is made available to the local unit even if it has not for the time being been directly involved in the care of the patient. Direct referrals may have little additional benefit for the patient; on the whole, they should be discouraged.

Service provision and performance of the specialist cardiac centre

Non-emergency investigation and treatment. The decision as to whether to proceed to surgery following invasive investigation may be surrendered to the specialist centre, or a case conference can be held there or at the district unit. Either way, except in exceptional circumstances, there is no indication for pre-operative assessment or follow-up review to be carried out elsewhere than in the district hospital, and all staff need to be briefed accordingly. Whether or not it is helpful for patients to attend the specialist centre for a single post-surgical follow-up is a matter of local practice.

The issue of waiting lists has become substantially muddied by purchaser/provider issues. The district health authority, acting as purchaser, must find some means of identifying a provider for the additional professional support needed by a district cardiological unit. The contracting process is likely to be cost sensitive and, in the long term, specific items of service are all likely to be priced. Average specialty costs will be crude and will reflect cost inflation by services that can be provided locally. In the shorter term, block contracts are based on historical arrangements, and later cost and volume contracts are likely to be in place. In general terms, target delays for routine invasive investigation should not exceed six weeks, whereas surgical or angioplasty intervention should not exceed three months; emergency admission for either should be within 24 hours.

Under the new arrangements, district health authorities (but not the district cardiologist) are making a guess as to the level of service provision required. Sometimes the specialist centres fulfil the work that they have contracted to undertake before the end of the financial year. They then face the difficult decision as to whether to overperform on their contract, and lose money, or to stop activity altogether.

Districts will vary in the amount of revenue set aside for extra contractual referrals representing capricious requests by non-fundholding general practitioners, or activity outside the basic contracts. Present governmental policies are that budgetary decisions have to be made at local level in a health service that is generally considered to be underfunded.[3] High cost interventions such as cardiac surgery are relatively unattractive, and they may become relatively less available to those who do not carry private health insurance.

Emergency investigation and treatment. During the years 1979–84, at St Peter's Hospital no less than 25% of all patients referred to the regional specialist centre suffered recent onset or unstable symptoms of angina pectoris requiring urgent revascularisation.[12] This comparatively high percentage fell to 17% over the full ten-year period,[13] and more patients were referred for coronary angiography with stable symptoms. An emergency referral to some extent dislocates the normal working of a cardiac department, and is more costly. It is thus essential that all such referrals should be made by a consultant, and preferably the consultant cardiologist at a district unit. In this way, a specialist centre may have confidence that the patients are appropriately referred and assessed. Such referrals are likely to be made only after there has been a failure of full medical treatment, and should expect to have a target transfer waiting time not exceeding 24 hours. This applies to permanent endocardial pacemaking, other haemodynamic upsets requiring urgent surgical intervention (such as ruptured chordae of the mitral valve and perforated intraventricular septum), and for emergency investigation or surgery in the acute coronary syndromes.

Queue jumping. Since the NHS and Community Care Act 1990, services increasingly are seen in part as a commercial transaction. One of the more surprising aspects of the fundholding process was that fundholders, notably general practitioners, have bought advantage for their patients in terms of shorter waiting times. This has led to discussions about the ethics of slow and fast track waiting list patients for surgery, with the former not prejudicing the latter if the activity is 'extra' to the routine work of the department. Queue jumping on the basis of ability to pay is now widespread and may represent the only means of survival for certain hardpressed district hospitals.[15] Once a patient requires surgery to improve his prognosis in the context of coronary heart disease, then the longer the wait and the greater the risk of mishap before he comes to surgery.

Communication

Good communication is an intrinsic part of patient care, but good organisation costs money. Often NHS staff have to work with inadequate information systems, in a poor environment. Secretarial and other administrative staff are overworked. Repeated 'efficiency' clawbacks by central government and recurring financial crises within Trusts and Directly Managed Units have generated an environment in which freezing of posts occurs without thought of the sometimes overwhelming burden that falls on those who provide the infrastructure on which clinical care is based. Modern technology, including word-processing, assisted by computerised patient records and electronic mail should make communication between district cardiologist, general practitioner and specialist cardiac centre prompt and effective.

Waiting list deaths

If there are delays in treatment, deaths will occur amongst patients who have to wait for treatment. The issue of deaths on the waiting list has been examined.[13,16] Over a ten-year period, 20 patients from St Peter's Hospital were identified as having died from a cardiovascular cause while on waiting lists for investigation or surgery. A total of 1,000 patients was referred for revascularisation or valvar surgery during this period. Thus 2% died on the waiting list, a figure similar to that of overall surgical mortality. At a time when health care is rationed, a close audit of the progress of individual patients based on the severity of their condition needs to be maintained with the regional centre. Waiting list policy at the specialist cardiac centre should be agreed with the purchaser and be freely accessible.

Research

Patients with coronary heart disease are not infrequently invited to take part in research programmes. Sometimes these research projects involve basic research and may be onerous; sometimes they are pharmaceutical trials which involve multiple attendances. Often the patients from the district centre have to travel a substantial distance to reach the specialist centre. Patients invited to take part in such programmes often do so on the basis that it might help them or others. In spite of careful briefing, it is likely that many only have a hazy notion as to what are the objectives of the enterprise, and what are the potential benefits. Academic units in particular have a requirement often for significant numbers of patients to support an active programme of research, often involving both regional trainees and visiting fellows.

It is as well for the local specialist to be involved if patients are being invited by regional centres to participate in research or in trials. Some patients have been upset by requests from a specialist centre that they enter research studies, and in one case a patient decided not to proceed with planned surgery. Consideration could be given to bilateral ethical review of any such research proposals.

Conclusion

There is an ongoing and substantial shortfall between the need and availability for cardiological services at all levels in the United Kingdom. This gap has closed somewhat in recent years but remains substantial. District general hospitals should be able to provide a full range of inpatient and outpatient services, that is apart from cardiac catheterisation (usually), cardiac surgery and coronary angioplasty.

Specialist cardiac centres should provide only those items of service specifically requested, and these should be carried out by designated operators.

The waiting list for routine investigation and revascularisation procedures should not exceed six weeks and three months respectively, while emergency investigation and surgery should be available within 24 hours. Longer delays have been demonstrated to be associated with increased morbidity and mortality.

It should be the responsibility of the district cardiologist to make all referrals for the uptake of specialist cardiac services on behalf of his/her hospital, having reached agreement with the purchasing authority. Non-specialists should not have direct access to these scarce and expensive services.

Prompt communication, using modern methods, is to be advocated, and catheter reports and surgical reports should be available within three working days of any procedure. Communication between district cardiologist, general practitioner and specialist cardiac centre must be prompt and effective.

References

1. Chamberlain DA, Goodwin JF, Emanuel RW, Bailey LG. Career prospects in cardiology in England and Wales: serving 15 health districts. *British Heart Journal* 1981; **45**: 46033.
2. Royal College of Physicians of London and Royal College of Surgeons of England. Combined cardiac centres for investigation and treatment with a note on the requirement of cardiology in hospitals outside such a centre: second joint report. *British Heart Journal* 1980; **43**: 211–9.
3. *Healthcare systems in transition.* Paris: OECD, 1990.
4. Chamberlain D, Bailey L, Emmanuel R, Oliver M. Staffing and facilities in cardiology in England and Wales July 1982: second biannual survey. *British Heart Journal* 1985; **50**: 597–604.
5. Chamberlain D, Bailey L, Julian D. Staffing and facilities in cardiology in the United Kingdom 1984: third biannual survey. *British Heart Journal* 1986; **55**: 311–20.
6. Chamberlain D, Bailey L, Southam E *et al.* Staffing in cardiology in the United Kingdom 1988: fifth biannual survey. *British Heart Journal* 1989; **62**: 482–7.
7. Chamberlain D, Pentecost D, Reval K *et al.* Staffing in cardiology in the United Kingdom 1990: sixth biannual survey, with data on facilities on cardiology in England and Wales 1989. *British Heart Journal* 1991; **66**: 395–404.
8. British Cardiac Society. Cardiology in the district hospital: report of a working group. *British Heart Journal* 1987; **58**: 537–46.
9. Joy M, Hugget I. Cardiology in the District Hospital. *British Medical Journal* 1982; **285**: 790–2.
10. National Health Service. *Coronary heart disease.* National Audit Office, London: HMSO, 1989.
11. Clinical Standards Advisory Group. *Access and availability of coronary artery bypass grafting and coronary angioplasty.* London: HMSO, 1993.

12. Cripps T, Dennis MS, Joy M. The need for invasive cardiological assessment and operations: viewpoint of a district general hospital. *British Heart Journal* 1986; **55**: 488–93

13. McRea CA, Marber MS, Keywood C, Joy M. The need for invasive cardiological assessment and intervention: a ten year review. *British Heart Journal* 1992; **67**: 200–3.

14. RITA trial participants. Coronary angioplasty versus coronary artery bypass surgery: the Randomised Intervention in the Treatment of Angina (RITA) trial. *Lancet* 1993; **341**: 573–80.

15. Joy M. The cost of hospital queue-jumping. *The Independent.* London, 15 May 1991.

16. Marber M, MacRae C, Joy M. Delay to invasive investigations and revascularisation for coronary heart disease in South West Thames region: a two tier system? *British Medical Journal* 1991; **302**: 1189–91.

11 | What happens in a specialist cardiac centre

David de Bono

Professor of Cardiology, University of Leicester

Cardiological practice in the United Kingdom has, for historical reasons, evolved a pyramidal structure whereby general practitioners have tended to refer patients to district general hospital physicians, who in turn refer selected patients to cardiologists working in specialist cardiac centres. There is evidence that a rigid referral hierarchy is breaking down, with many general practitioners now referring patients direct to cardiologists, whilst many cardiac centres, particularly those outside London, also have a more or less explicit 'district general hospital' role. Some of the advantages and disadvantages of direct referral and of 'filtered' referral through a district general hospital physician are listed in Table 1.

The topic is discussed in more detail in the preceding chapter. The services that a specialist referral centre would normally offer are listed in Table 2. Those of most relevance to the management of chest pain are the cardiac catheter laboratory, direct access to

Table 1. Comparison of direct referral to a specialist cardiac centre with that through a district hospital.

Type of referral	Advantages	Disadvantages
Direct GP referral	Rapid access at time of highest patient risk	Risk of blocking clinics with trivial referrals
	Simplifies long-term shared care with GP	Potentially wasteful of expensive resource
Referral through general physician with interest in cardiology	Ensures selection of appropriate cases	May waste valuable time
	Simplifies resource management	Places responsibility on physician to remain up to date
	May provide hospital back-up closer to home	

Table 2. Facilities provided.

District hospital	Specialist centre
Physician with an interest	Specialist cardiologists
Exercise testing	Exercise testing
Echocardiography	Sophisticated echocardiography
(Radionuclide studies)	Radionuclide studies
	Coronary angiography/PTCA
	Coronary surgery

coronary angioplasty and coronary artery surgery, and perhaps access to more sophisticated radionuclide facilities than are available at most district general hospitals.

The decision-making process in a specialist cardiac centre is

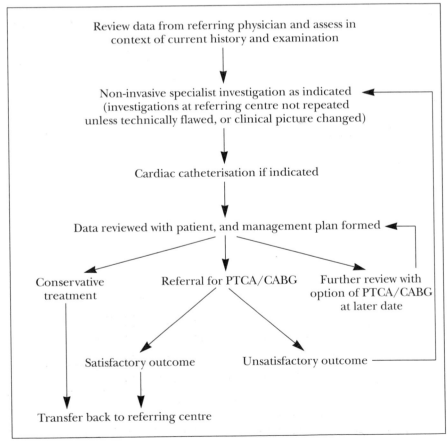

Fig. 1. *Decision-making process in a specialist cardiac centre.*

summarised in Fig. 1. Ideally, all patients referred to such a centre should be suitable for, and should go on to receive the benefit of, the specialist diagnostic facilities in the specialist centre. This is normally the case for patients referred from physicians with a special interest and training in cardiology, and indeed many specialist cardiac centres have arrangements whereby physicians with an interest from neighbouring district hospitals have sessional contracts and full access to the investigative facilities. The referral match may be less perfect for other physicians, and agreed referral policies may be helpful. Patient symptoms may change, for better or worse, fairly rapidly, and this may change appropriate management when the patient arrives at the specialist cardiac centre.

In order to explore more fully the work of a specialist cardiac centre, I shall discuss an audit of 767 consecutive outpatient referrals to a single cardiology clinic between June 1989 and May 1990. The centre receives referrals both from general practitioners and from general physicians in the local university teaching hospitals and in neighbouring district general hospitals.

New outpatients were logged by the doctor at the time of clinic attendance using a simple data input form. All patients were followed up over a one-year period in terms of their utilisation of exercise testing, cardiac catheterisation, angioplasty and cardiac surgery.

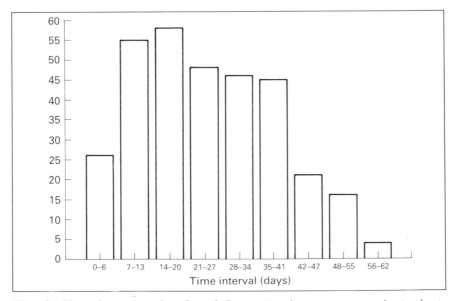

Fig. 2. *Time between referral and first outpatient assessment in patients with a working diagnosis of ischaemic heart disease.*

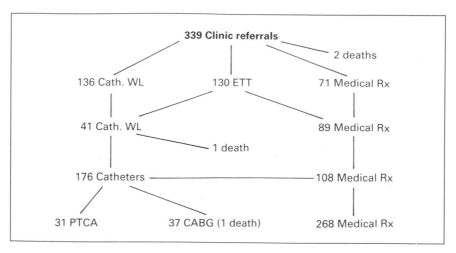

Fig. 3. *Pattern of investigation in patients with a working diagnosis of ischaemic heart disease.* Cath. WL = Catheter WL; ETT = exercise tolerance test; PTCA = coronary angioplasty; CABG = coronary artery bypass graft surgery.

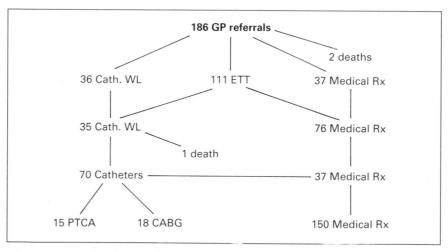

Fig. 4. *Investigation and outcome in patients referred direct from general practitioners.*

There were 367 referrals with a working diagnosis of ischaemic heart disease out of 767 referrals. Data on the source of referral were missing on 28 patients. There were 186 referrals (55%) from general practitioners, and 153 (45%) from other physicians. Mean age was 57.8 years and the age distribution of general practitioner and hospital consultant referrals was similar; 104 patients (28.3%) were aged 65 or over.

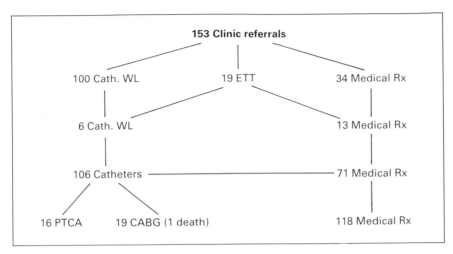

Fig. 5. *Investigation and outcome in patients from other consultant clinics.*

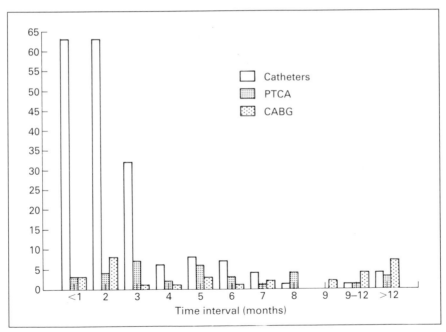

Fig. 6. *Time interval between first clinic appointment and coronary arteriography, angioplasty and coronary bypass grafting.*

The median waiting time between the date of the referral letter and the date of first clinic attendance was 26 days (range 1–62 days) (Fig. 2). Waiting times did not differ significantly between referrals from general practitioners and from other hospital physicians.

The outcome of referral for all patients with 'ischaemic heart disease' is shown in Fig. 3, and for patients referred by general practitioners and by hospital consultants separately in Figs 4 and 5. Eighteen percent of general practitioner referrals and 22% of consultant referrals eventually resulted in angioplasty (PTCA) or coronary bypass grafting (CABG). The proportion of angiograms that resulted in PTCA was 18%; by comparison, in the Confidential Enquiry into the Complications of Coronary Catheterisation (CECCC) study[1] the proportion was 15.8% for those centres carrying out both diagnostic angiography and PTCA. The proportion of patients aged 65 or over who underwent PTCA or CABG was similar to that for younger patients.

The timing of cardiac catheterisation, angioplasty and coronary bypass surgery is shown in Fig. 6. Half the catheter studies were done within 6 weeks of first clinic attendance. There was a wide range of intervals between first clinic attendance and PTCA or CABG.

During the period of the audit, two patients died after referral by their general practitioner but before their first clinic attendance, one patient died between having an exercise test and being admitted for a catheter study, no patient died while on the waiting list for surgery but one had a non-fatal infarct, and one patient died after surgery.

This is a description of experience at one centre; no claim is made that it is representative of the United Kingdom as a whole. Clearly those referred do not reflect the population age distribution of ischaemic heart disease (Chapters 2 and 3), but have been filtered by a combination of self-assessment and general practitioner assessment. The differences in pattern of investigation between referrals from general practitioners and district general hospital physicians illustrated in Figs 4 and 5 arise largely because most patients of the latter have already had exercise tests at their local hospital. The similarities in intervention rate between general practitioner initiated and consultant initiated referrals may conceal important differences in 'case mix'; for example, patients whose ischaemic heart disease presents with myocardial infarction are usually admitted in the first instance to a district general hospital, and constitute a substantial proportion of those subsequently referred to a specialist cardiac centre for advice about angina.

'Waiting lists' may have some validity with respect to outpatient appointments and initial catheter investigation, but become meaningless when considering coronary bypass grafting or angioplasty. Ideally, if a procedure needs to be done it should be done as soon as possible. In practice, some patients, presumably those with severe symptoms and coronary lesions of a type judged to put the patient at particular risk, have surgery very early; others are deferred for periods of up to one year. That no patients died on our surgical waiting list, and only 2% in the study reported by Joy in the preceding chapter, shows that cardiologists and cardiac surgeons have some skill in ranking patients in order of priority. However, this ranking is not infallible, and an imbalance between demand for and provision of surgical services may make it difficult to operate.

Reference

1   de Bono DP (on behalf of the Joint Audit Committee of the British Cardiac Society and the Royal College of Physicians of London). Complications of diagnostic cardiac catheterisation: results from 34,041 patients in the United Kingdom confidential enquiry into cardiac catheter complications. *British Heart Journal* 1993; **70**: 297–300.

12 | Differences in referral patterns for coronary angiography in one health region in the UK

David Gray
*Senior Lecturer in Medicine and Honorary Consultant Physician,
University Hospital, Nottingham*

The use of coronary angiography in the management of ischaemic heart disease varies widely. In the United States about three times as many procedures per million population are carried out as in the United Kingdom,[1] and in Canada more than twice as many,[2] but even within the USA the number of procedures differs from one state to another.[3]

In 1986 a target rate of 300 coronary artery bypass operations per million population was proposed, but there was no recommendation as to who should be investigated.[4] In 1989 we assembled an expert panel of doctors involved in the clinical care and investigation of patients with ischaemic heart disease to rate hypothetical 'indications' (or clinical scenarios) for coronary angiography; we then reviewed the notes of patients who had recently had angiography, and applied the panel's ratings of the *hypothetical* indicators to the *actual* patients to get a measure of 'appropriateness' for each clinical case.[5] We found that the degree of appropriateness of the procedure differed markedly between the three designated cardiac investigation centres in the Trent region, one of fourteen health regions in the UK (Table 1).

Centre 1, with ratings least in agreement with the consensus

Table 1. Degree of 'appropriateness' (%) of coronary angiography in the three cardiac centres in Trent region.

	Appropriate	Equivocal	Inappropriate
Centre 1	37	36	27
Centre 2	46	26	28
Centre 3	63	27	10

panel, was Sheffield; centre 2 was Leicester and centre 3, with ratings nearest to those of the panel, was Nottingham. Being considered 'appropriate' does not necessarily mean that the decision to
investigate was 'correct', nor does an 'inappropriate' rating mean
that the decision was 'wrong'—a different panel might have produced slightly different ratings, and the limited data from clinical
trials upon which doctors currently base their clinical decisions was
derived from selected populations which are probably not representative of the wide range of patients who appear in hospital clinics.

This study led us to believe that the process to select patients
with suspected myocardial ischaemia for cardiac catheterisation
may vary across the region. A more comprehensive study of all
patients undergoing invasive investigation in our region was undertaken first to establish whether different sorts of patients were
being referred for coronary angiography, and second to ascertain
the outcome of the investigation.

Method

Data were collected prospectively from all patients undergoing
coronary angiography in the three regional centres at Sheffield,
Leicester and Nottingham by research assistants participating in
the British Cardiac Society Randomised Intervention Treatment of
Angina (RITA) study, the results of which have been published.[6]
Data from RITA were supplemented by detailed information in the
patient record at or shortly after the catheter procedure. The
notes of all patients undergoing coronary angiography between
1 July 1988 and 30 June 1989 were reviewed.

Patients were identified according to their home address postcode as being resident within the cities of Sheffield, Leicester or
Nottingham, or in other urban or rural areas within the Trent
region. Patients who were resident outside the local health
authority were excluded from study. All patients were followed for
at least one year after the cardiac catheterisation. In some cases
data were incomplete, but there was a core of information available
for all patients for analysis.

Patient demography

During the data collection period, 2,096 cardiac catheterisations
were performed in the three regional referral centres for cardiac
catheterisation. Sheffield performed 699 procedures, Leicester
1,001 and Nottingham 396. Of these, 636 were excluded from the

analysis—432 catheters were arranged primarily to investigate valvular disorders; 156 to assess diverse conditions including congenital heart disease, cardiomyopathy and assessment for cardiac transplantation; and 48 patients had been referred from outside the Trent region.

The remaining 1,460 procedures were carried out to investigate symptoms suggestive of ischaemic heart disease; during the data collection period, 480 eligible cardiac catheterisations were performed in Sheffield, 729 in Leicester and 251 in Nottingham.

Each centre investigated all (or nearly all) patients from its own city (Fig. 1), and there was a flow of patients across county borders (Fig. 2), with almost all patients from South Yorkshire referred to Sheffield and almost all from Leicestershire to Leicester for investigation. Leicester also looked after most of the patients from Nottinghamshire and other areas which included Derby and Lincolnshire.

The ratio of men to women was 4.3 in Sheffield, 3.4 in Leicester and 3.2 in Nottingham. The age distribution of patients investigated in each centre, shown in Fig. 3, was similar in all centres, with few patients under the age of 40 and very few over the age of 80. The mean age was 54 years in Sheffield, 55 in Nottingham and 56

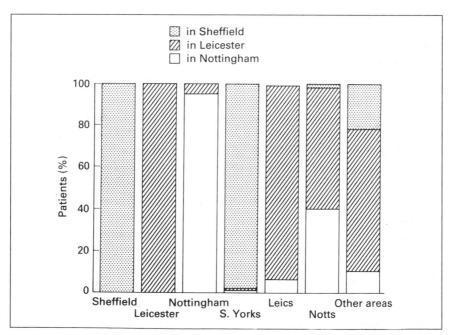

Fig. 1. *Coronary angiography in the Trent regional centres: where patients resided (according to postcode) and where they were investigated.*

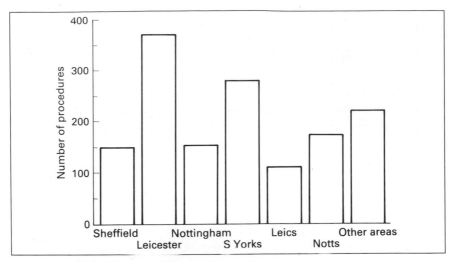

Fig. 2. *Areas of residence of patients.*

in Leicester. The distribution of ages of patients referred from outside a regional centre from other hospitals was similar to that of
patients locally resident, but the ratio of men to women was the
same at 3.8 for each centre.

The most frequently documented reason for carrying out

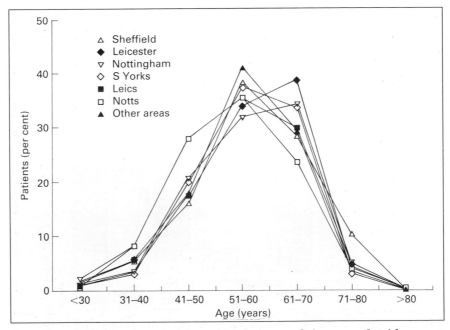

Fig. 3. *Age distribution of patients in relation to their areas of residence.*

Table 2. Reasons for coronary angiography, variations in drugs employed before angiography, and results of exercise testing in some specialist cardiac centres.

	Sheffield	Leicester	Nottingham	S Yorks	Leics	Notts	Other
Reasons for angiography							
Angina	147	340	148	274	98	162	211
Post-myocardial infarction	3	31	6	6	12	12	10
Persistent pain	116	287	129	213	84	143	182
(%)	79	84	87	78	86	88	86
Previous myocardial infarction	62	169	83	128	45	85	105
(%)	50	52	63	57	47	55	54
Unstable angina	31	27	16	25	4	10	25
(%)	25	8	12	13	4	6	13
Drugs employed before angiography							
Beta-antagonist	86	248	120	182	75	134	173
(%)	59	73	81	65	68	77	78
Long-acting nitrate	94	180	105	167	66	115	160
(%)	64	53	71	60	60	66	72
Calcium antagonist	94	160	118	189	52	114	172
(%)	64	47	80	68	47	47	78
Exercise testing							
Results positive at an early stage	44	108	64	137	29	87	42
(%)	38	32	43	50	31	50	20

Table 3. Principal findings on coronary angiography in some specialist cardiac centres.

	Sheffield	Leicester	Nottingham	S Yorks	Leics	Notts	Other
Normal angiogram	27	45	22	54	15	18	26
(%)	18	12	14	19	14	10	12
Left main stem lesion	13	40	11	18	13	16	21
(%)	9	12	7	5	12	9	10
Prox. left anterior descending lesion	60	171	76	107	48	79	103
(%)	40	46	49	38	44	45	47
Left ventricular function impairment (%):							
severe	3(2)	26(7)	12(8)	0(0)	3(3)	14(8)	6(13)
mod/mild	61(41)	164(44)	34(22)	135(48)	57(52)	61(35)	111(50)
normal	86(57)	178(48)	102(69)	143(52)	50(45)	99(57)	104(47)

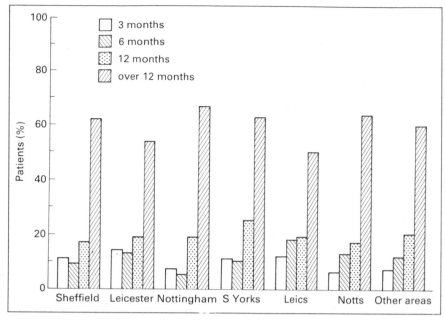

Fig. 4. *Duration of symptoms before coronary angiography.*

angiography in all patients in this study was to investigate chest pain which was thought to be due to angina, with only a few being investigated in the recovery phase of an *acute* myocardial infarction (Table 2). Most patients had persistent angina despite medication when presenting for angiography. One-eighth of patients from Leicester and Leicestershire were apparently free from angina at the time of cardiac catheterisation, at least twice as many as from other cities and districts (Table 2).

The duration of chest pain symptoms ranged from one month to over one year (Fig. 4); over 80% of patients had had symptoms for at least six months, and two-thirds for more than twelve months before having cardiac catheterisation. Fewer patients from Leicester had long-standing symptoms compared with the other cities; patients from Leicestershire generally had symptoms of shorter duration than patients from South Yorkshire, Nottinghamshire and the other areas.

Pre-catheter events

Previous myocardial infarction was a common finding in patients from all areas. Two-thirds of patients from Nottingham had sustained a myocardial infarction prior to catheterisation compared

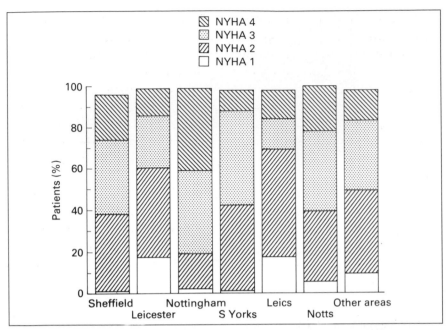

Fig. 5. *Severity of symptoms on the New York Heart Association scale.*

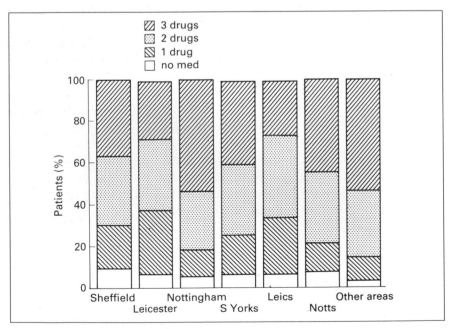

Fig. 6. *Drug prescribing.*

with about half from Leicester and Sheffield (Table 2). Slightly more than half of the patients from South Yorkshire, Nottinghamshire and other areas had had a myocardial infarction, and slightly less than half from Leicestershire (Table 2).

In the six months prior to angiography, 145 patients (22% of all patients) had had an episode of unstable angina. Of these, 65% had a cardiac catheter during the acute admission with unstable symptoms. Sheffield doctors were more likely than the other centres to arrange a catheter during the acute admission for their patients (Table 2).

Severity of symptoms, according to the New York Heart Association criteria, showed that more Nottingham patients had symptoms of severe angina than patients from Sheffield or Leicester (Fig. 5). Patients from Leicestershire had generally milder symptoms than those from South Yorkshire, Nottinghamshire or the other areas.

Pre-catheter medication

Medication to control symptoms before catheterisation had been used extensively. Overall, only 6% of patients were on no regular medication at all at the time of the cardiac catheter, 21% of patients were taking at least one drug to control symptoms, 27% at least two and 36% three types of drug (Fig. 6). A few were taking a diuretic in addition. Patients from Leicester and Leicestershire were taking fewer tablets than patients elsewhere. Patients from Nottingham, Nottinghamshire and other areas were more likely to be taking several drugs.

Prescribing preferences were apparent in the three centres (Table 2). The most frequently prescribed agent, taken by almost three-quarters of all patients, was a beta-antagonist, followed by a long-acting nitrate and a calcium antagonist. Beta-antagonists were used preferentially by patients from all areas except Sheffield and South Yorkshire, where calcium antagonists predominated. As a second agent, Leicester and Leicestershire patients had a long-acting nitrate, while Nottingham, Nottinghamshire and the other areas had a calcium antagonist.

Pre-catheter investigations

An exercise test prior to catheterisation was carried out by about two-thirds of all patients, using either the Sheffield or the Bruce protocol. Tests were performed on 69% of patients from Leicester,

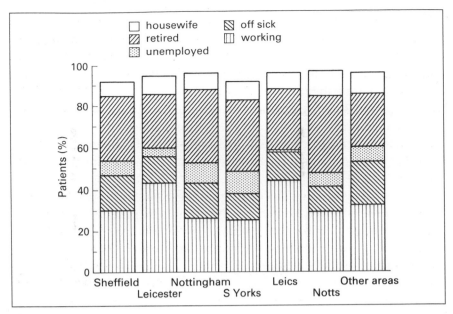

Fig. 7. *Employment status.*

65% from Nottingham and 30% from Sheffield; where tests were carried out, these were positive in 68% of those done in Leicester, 75% in Nottingham and 74% in Sheffield. Exercise testing in peripheral hospitals showed a similar pattern; fewer were done in South Yorkshire (42%) than in Leicestershire (71%), Nottinghamshire (72%) and other areas (74%), with a high positive rate in all areas (Table 2).

Nottingham patients frequently had tests considered positive at an early stage (Table 2). Patients who had exercise tests performed in Leicester, Leicestershire and Sheffield usually managed to exceed stage 1 of a Bruce protocol (or equivalent performance using the Sheffield protocol), while the majority of the remaining patients failed to reach this standard.

Exercise thallium-201, methylisobutyl isonitrile (MIBI) and multiple-gated analysis (MUGA) tests were carried out on less than 1% of all patients.

The employment status of patients is shown in Fig. 7; overall, 34% of patients were in regular employment, 15% were off work due to ill health and 40% were retired, more than one-third of them on health grounds. Patients from Leicester and Leicestershire were more likely to be in work than patients from elsewhere.

Overall, 5% of patients held either a heavy goods or public service vehicle or pilot's licence at the time of catheterisation.

Findings at angiography

Coronary artery bypass surgery (CABG) had already been carried out in 8% of patients from Sheffield, 10% from Leicester, 5% from Nottingham and 6% from outside referral centres. Previous percutaneous coronary angioplasty (PTCA) had been performed on 6% of Sheffield patients, 5% from Leicester, 1% from Nottingham and 4% from elsewhere.

Fourteen percent of *all* coronary angiograms did not show surgically significant coronary artery disease (Table 3). More patients from Sheffield and South Yorkshire were thought to have a normal angiogram than patients from elsewhere. Three-vessel disease was found in over half the patients from Nottingham and 42% from Sheffield and Leicester; significant left main stem disease was found in 11% of all patients, and proximal left anterior descending artery lesions were found in 51% of all patients (Table 3).

Left ventricular function is shown in Table 3. Severe dysfunction was found in 5% of all patients.

Management

The management options available following this series of cardiac catheterisations were elective coronary artery bypass surgery or elective percutaneous transluminal coronary angioplasty, randomisation to either surgery or angioplasty (as part of the RITA study)

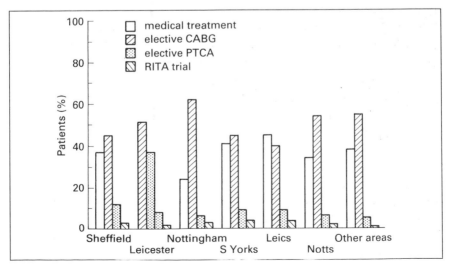

Fig. 8. *Planned management.*

or continued medical treatment. Overall, 46% of patients were referred for elective CABG, 8% for elective PTCA and 41% were managed medically (Fig. 8). Patients catheterised in Sheffield and Nottingham were more likely to proceed to a revascularisation procedure than to continue medical management, but this was not so for patients investigated in Leicester.

In 3% of patients, the chances of successful revascularisation by either CABG or PTCA were thought to be the same, so these patients were randomised in the RITA trial.[6]

Discussion

A good history, physical examination and non-invasive and invasive tests yield information which is of diagnostic and prognostic value,[7] but only coronary angiography can define suitability for coronary revascularisation. Once the coronary anatomy is known, decision-making *may* become easier despite slightly conflicting results from the major trials.[8-10] Coronary artery bypass surgery should be offered in place of medical treatment to patients with greater than 50% luminal narrowing of the left main stem, three-vessel disease with impaired left ventricular function and probably also to those with significant narrowing of the proximal left anterior descending artery. PTCA was not available at the time of these cited trials but the value of PTCA was assessed in the RITA trial,[6] where patients in whom equivalent revascularisation was thought achievable by either surgery or angioplasty were randomised to CABG or PTCA, with follow-up to 5 years planned. After 2.5 years, both techniques of revascularisation were associated with similar risk of death or reinfarction, but patients who had CABG enjoyed better relief of angina, while those who had PTCA were more likely to complain of symptoms and to have had a repeat attempt at myocardial revascularisation.

The indications for coronary angiography are still 'unsettled',[11] but in stable angina they fall into three categories. First, it may be performed to confirm clinically suspected coronary artery disease (as a prelude to bypass surgery); second, to stratify risk for prognostic purposes; and third, to obtain an accurate diagnosis where other investigations have failed. The variation in practice revealed by this study suggests that consideration that a patient is suitable for angiography probably depends on the philosophy and style of practice of the clinician: those who seek to control symptoms may persist with escalating doses of up to three drugs until symptoms cannot be controlled with medication; those who are concerned about minimising risk can justify angiography at a much earlier stage to avoid missing patients with left main stem disease or significant extensive coronary disease. All cardiologists will see patients with an indeterminate diagnosis despite extensive tests for non-cardiac causes.

This spectrum of clinical activity in relation to invasive investigation is seen in the Trent region survey, with apparent polarisation towards symptomatic control in Nottingham and avoidance of risk in Leicester and Sheffield.

It should be stressed that for most patients the investigation of coronary angiography led to intervention with either coronary surgery or angioplasty. The long duration of symptoms suffered by most patients before angiography is probably sufficient evidence that most cardiac catheter procedures were carried out to determine the extent of disease and subsequent suitability for surgery.

The patients from Nottingham had advanced ischaemic heart disease at the time of angiography. They tended to have symptoms for a longer time than most; most had angina graded moderately severe or severe on New York Heart Association criteria, they were more likely to have had a myocardial infarction at some time, they required extensive drug treatment to limit symptoms, they frequently had early positive stress tests, significant coronary lesions were common at cardiac catheter, and most were accepted for either coronary artery bypass surgery or angioplasty.

Leicester patients seemed to have milder degrees of coronary disease. For most patients symptoms were of shorter duration, angina was less severe, and more had no pain when admitted for cardiac catheterisation, fewer patients had two or three drugs to control symptoms, patients were more likely to hold down a job, and performance on treadmill testing was somewhat better than for most. Investigation of these patients with milder symptoms did not increase the rate at which a normal coronary angiogram was found. Leicester had a low rate compared with other centres; significant coronary lesions were as likely to be found. However, only half were recommended for further intervention. The distal vasculature may have been considered unsuitable or milder symptoms may have precluded surgery or angioplasty.

Sheffield patients appear to have milder disease than those from Nottingham and more severe than those from Leicester. Non-invasive investigation was used less frequently to assess patients with chronic stable angina, and this may have been responsible for the increased proportion of normal coronary arteries seen.

The Leicester approach of obtaining an angiogram at an earlier stage in the disease process was more successful in identifying patients with significant disease of the left main stem than that in the other centres. The Nottingham approach of checking an angiogram later in the disease process suffers from a lack of knowledge of which patients who have *not* had a catheter and have mild symptoms only are being denied access to surgery of proven benefit. Also, there may have been some patients with left main stem disease who died without referral for coronary angiography.

The only other major difference between the regional catheter centres at Sheffield and Leicester and all other hospitals (including Nottingham) was the increased chance of having angiography during an admission with unstable angina. This may be due to differences in philosophy or simply in organisation: Sheffield and Leicester have facilities for angioplasty and surgery, while Nottingham can offer neither of these.

Patients referred to regional centres tended to be similar to those of the centres themselves; comparison is easiest in South Yorkshire and Leicestershire where cross-border flow was minimal. The drug treatment profile was similar, as was symptom severity and duration, and the use of exercise testing. This presumably reflects local knowledge of, and general acceptance of, the expectations of the receiving unit.

Our initial impression that there were differences in the referral patterns for coronary angiography in the Trent region appears to have been upheld, with angiography being used by some as a diagnostic test and by others as a prognostic indicator. Although both approaches are valid (showing in this study the ability to detect coronary artery disease), reliance on symptoms can be limiting. Symptoms do not correlate closely with the extent of coronary disease,[12] and the recognised benefits of bypass surgery with respect to mortality may be denied to patients with severe coronary disease.

The survey of all patients on nitrates reviewed by John Hampton in Chapter 3 showed that the general practitioner acted as a gatekeeper, controlling access to cardiology, treating at least fifteen patients with angina for each one known to the hospital.[13]

A strategy for adequate evaluation of *all* patients with coronary artery disease, which combines both prognostic and diagnostic aspects of invasive cardiology, might be possible in the Trent region but the prospect is daunting.

The 'hidden' number of angina patients in the Trent region could lead to a large rise in the number of invasive investigations being requested, should there be even a small change in referral pattern by the general practitioners or in the working practices of hospital physicians and cardiologists. It would not be practicable to undertake coronary angiography on every patient. We need to select patients for coronary angiography (whether for diagnosis or prognosis) by applying stricter criteria based on recognised non-invasive indicators of prognosis using exercise tests[14] (Chapter 5) and thallium scanning,[7] risking missing some patients with life-threatening coronary disease. We also need more probability analysis,[15] priority assessment[2] or a pre-test assessment[16] of the influence of the result of coronary angiography on further management.

References

1. National Centre for Health Statistics. National hospital discharge survey. Annual summary, United States, 1987. *Vital and health statistics.* Series 13. No. 99. DHHS publication (PHS) 89-1760. Washington, DC: Government Printing Office, 1989.

2. Naylor CD, Baigrie RS, Goldman BS, Basinski A. Assessment of priority for coronary revascularisation procedure. *Lancet* 1990; **i**: 1070–3.

3. Chassin MR, Kosecoff J, Park RE, Fink AR, Rauchman S, Keesey J, Flynn MF, Brook RH. Variations in the use of medical and surgical services by the Medicare population. *New England Journal of Medicine* 1986; **314**: 285–90.

4. UK Consensus Development Conference. Coronary artery bypass surgery: a consensus. *Lancet* 1984; **ii**: 1269.

5. Gray D, Hampton JR, Bernstein SJ, Kocekoff J, Brook RH. Audit of coronary angiography and bypass surgery. *Lancet* 1990; **335**: 1317–20.

6. RITA participants. Coronary angioplasty versus coronary artery bypass surgery: the Randomised Intervention Trial of Angina (RITA). *Lancet* 1993; **341**: 573–80.

7. Bobbio M, Pollock BH, Cohen I, Diamond GA. Comparative accuracy of clinical tests for diagnosis and prognosis of coronary artery disease. *American Journal of Cardiology* 1988; **62**: 896–900.

8. CASS principal investigators and their associates. Coronary Artery Surgery Study (CASS): a randomised trial of coronary artery bypass surgery. Survival data. *Circulation* 1983; **68**: 939–50.

9. European Coronary Surgery Group. Longterm results of coronary artery bypass surgery in stable angina pectoris. *Lancet* 1982; **ii**:1173–80.

10. Detre K, Hultgren H, Takaro T. Veterans Administration cooperative study of surgery for coronary arterial occlusive disease. III. Methods and baseline characteristics, including experience with medical treatment. *American Journal of Cardiology* 1977; **40**: 212–25.

11. Ambrose JA. Unsettled indications for coronary angiography. *Journal of the American College of Cardiology* 1984; **3**: 1575–80.

12. Bruscke AVG, Proudfit WL, Sones FM. Progress study of 590 consecutive nonsurgical cases of coronary disease followed 5–9 years: ventriculographic and other correlations. *Circulation* 1973; **47**: 1154–63.

13. Cannon PJ, Stockley IH, Connell PA, Garner ST, Hampton JR.

Prevalence of angina as assessed by a survey of nitrate prescriptions. *Lancet* 1988; **i**: 979–81.

14. Sanmarco ME, Pontius S, Selvester RH. Abnormal blood pressure response and marked ischaemic ST segment depression as predictors of severe coronary artery disease. *Circulation* 1980; **61**: 572–8.

15. Epstein SE. Implications of probability analysis on the strategy used for noninvasive detection of coronary artery disease: role of single or combined use of exercise electrocardiographic testing, radionuclide cineangiography and myocardial perfusion imaging. *American Journal of Cardiology* 1980; **46**: 491–9.

16. Knoebel SB. Treatment of coronary artery disease. *Journal of the American College of Cardiology* 1989; **13**: 957–68.

13 | Audit in cardiological practice

Peter Wilkinson
Consultant Physician, Ashford Hospital, Ashford, Middlesex

Attempts made to assess the quality of medical care in a systematic way were initiated by authors such as Donabedian in 1966 who described the concepts and the available tools,[1] but it was not until the early 1980s that this work began to filter into the clinical environment when groups of enthusiasts began to publish their experiences. The Royal College of Physicians has recently required that audit take place for medical posts to be approved for training purposes, and thus formal audit programmes of varying quality have been created in each hospital,[2,3] with specific guidance from the College.[4,5] This chapter will discuss the audit process and will suggest a variety of ways in which audit can be used to assess the management of the patient with suspected angina.

Background to clinical audit

The components of clinical audit are to observe practice, set a standard of practice, compare observed practice with the standard, implement change and observe practice after changes have been implemented (Fig. 1). The activity to be audited should be common,

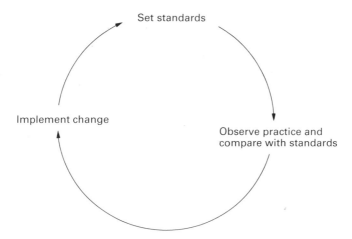

Fig. 1. *An audit cycle.*

and its effect on patients and resources important. In addition, the activity to be audited must be easily defined and assessed, standards for it must be capable of being agreed and defined, and the process of care should be amenable to change. The management of suspected angina fits most of these criteria, although whether standards can be agreed amongst all cardiologists is open to question, as previous chapters in this book indicate.

Clinical audit can play a major educational role by identifying a gap in knowledge, a problem in communication, or a need for acquisition or enhancement of particular knowledge or skills in a group or an individual.[6] Time and resources are needed to create a programme that can correct these deficiencies and, if it can be shown that as a result of this educational endeavour practice has changed, the audit cycle has been completed. Audit can also be used as a tool to highlight the need for a change in the way a department is managed or funded. Some sceptics doubt if audit will lead to change and need to be convinced that this investment in time, effort and money will have an effect on outcome, but if audit is conducted in a systematic manner[7] it can be effective in changing behaviour.[8] Those devising programmes aimed at enhancing education need to be aware that the needs of the doctors in the training grades and of consultants may be different. For example, doctors in training move around frequently, so audit needs to be a process of setting standards, assessing performance and feeding back the information gained within the span of their appointment.[9] There also needs to be a strategy that will include a regular review of common problems, such as suspected angina. Doctors in training should be involved in decisions about the format of the clinical audit programme.

Clinical audit in the new health care environment

Doctors have always been interested in the quality of care they provide, but there has been a tendency by the profession in the past to make the assumption that all care was appropriate and of the highest quality, without examining the evidence; the ability of the individual consultant to practise with complete clinical freedom went unchallenged. When doctors had little impact on clinical outcome, this attitude might not have been of any great consequence but, with the increasing technical complexity and cost of medicine, the purchasers of care want to ensure that their money is spent wisely, and the consumers of care that they are being offered the best possible quality of medicine. Research has aimed at pushing forward the frontiers of science rather than ensuring that the best available practices are in place throughout the country.

The separation of purchaser and provider of care in the UK results from the NHS and Community Care Act 1990. Doctors will find that purchasers want to test the appropriateness of care, and they will be examined critically since cardiology is perceived as an expensive specialty. Cardiologists should find an ally in their local Director of Public Health whose responsibility is to assess the health care needs of the population and to ensure that they are being met.

The power of general practice fundholders is starting to be felt. It is conceivable that they may retain patients with angina without referral to a cardiologist, in an attempt to save money for other clinical purposes. The patient's perception of the quality of care is also a suitable matter for audit.

Clinical audit takes place within hospitals and in general practice centres between fellow professionals who will have to maintain a spirit of openness in describing how they handle patients, so that mistakes come to be seen as opportunities to learn and to improve the future quality of care. This involves a change in professional attitudes which will have to be carefully nurtured.[10] The recent emphasis on the internal market and on maintaining a competitive environment may affect this spirit.

Using the information presented in the previous chapters, audit will be approached from each step as the patient moves upwards in the referral ladder.

The patient's perspective

One of the reasons why the profession should audit its activities is that, if it does not, someone from outside the profession will. However, even in the United States, where consumerism is rife, the role of the patient in the process of assessing the quality of health care remains uncertain.[11] The needs of patients with chest pain are clear—rapid assessment, appropriate treatment of high standard delivered with humanity, and the provision of sufficient information about their condition to enable them to share in decisions about treatment. Some of these elements are open to clinical audit, and cardiologists, like all physicians, should be intermittently surveying patients' satisfaction with the services they offer, including feedback on facilities offered and attitudes encountered.

When the quality of technical care is being assessed, patients usually have to leave this to their doctors as their professional

advocate. However, doctors, at whatever level in the chain of referral, should be aware of the strengths and weaknesses of colleagues
so that the most appropriate referral can be made.

The general practitioner

In Chapter 4, Dr Inman reveals many of the dilemmas facing a
general practitioner dealing with a patient who has suspected angina, whilst the evidence provided by Professor Hampton in Chapter
3 suggests that general practitioners are dealing with large numbers of patients with angina without referring them to a district
general hospital or regional cardiologist.

Should so many patients with angina be managed without an
outpatient referral, or should a standard be set that suggests that
every patient with possible angina should be referred for at least
one assessment by a consultant? If patients are being managed by a
general practitioner, the care received by a proportion should be
open to audit, preferably by a visiting consultant with an interest in
cardiology. At present the process of audit is usually separated into
hospital and general practice; this division needs to be broken
down. Guidelines could help set standards against which audit
could be conducted. These guidelines, developed locally from
national guidelines to suit local arrangements such as those outlined in Chapter 15, could suggest appropriate investigations in
someone with suspected angina, recommend treatment and guide
referral. The structure of the service available to cardiac patients
in general practice is auditable so, for example, a standard could
be set that a general practitioner should either have access to an
ECG machine or to a service provided in a local hospital without
the need to refer the patient to outpatients or to the accident and
emergency department. Those practices with a local formulary can
already audit their care relating to the use of agreed drugs.

General practitioners will also wish to know how many patients
they refer for a second opinion compared with colleagues, this
being particularly relevant to fundholders who may see referral as
an option with a price tag.

Referral from primary care

This referral is usually to a physician with an interest in cardiology
in a district general hospital, but it can be made directly to a cardiac centre if the general practitioner is near one (see Chapters 10
and 11). As a proportion of district hospitals in the UK do not have

a physician with an interest in cardiology, one immediate way to produce care of higher quality would be to appoint such a person in every district hospital.[12]

As pointed out by Dr Birkhead in Chapter 8, the facilities available at a district hospital should include access to 12 lead ECG, exercise ECG, echocardiography and ambulatory ECG. The British Cardiac Society has laid down what it expects to find in such a hospital, and its document can be used by purchasers when preparing contracts with competing providing units. However, there is no inspection system to ensure that the range of services is adequate. The British Cardiac Society might consider a regular inspection of hospitals along the lines pioneered by Dr Richard Wray in South East Thames region, using two visiting consultants, one from inside and one from outside the region. A report by external assessors may be more influential with managers in the creation of necessary improvements. These visits, if performed tactfully, also have the potential to comment on the way a department is run, pointing out possible areas for change, as well as highlighting innovative practices that could be used elsewhere. Suitable topics for audit include the appropriateness of referrals for consideration of angioplasty or surgery; a general practitioner could comment on feedback from patients about the care received in the hospital. In the USA these aspects of care are often left without comment, as the need to maintain referral patterns can stifle openness owing to the fear that patients might be referred elsewhere. This is true to a lesser extent in the UK, but purchasers are likely to take an increasing interest in the results of such audits. Referral patterns in private practice may also inhibit discussion about the appropriateness of referral.

Local guidelines must be developed within a hospital to enable standards to be set, against which audit can be conducted. The number and appropriateness of investigations used by individuals or teams of doctors can be audited, as can whether the results obtained were interpreted correctly. It is no good blaming colleagues for abusing a service if guidelines for its use have not been clearly delineated within a hospital. Chapter 5 by Dr Irving reveals some of the flaws in exercise ECG testing, suggesting that a useful audit exercise would be to examine the indications for exercise tests, the interpretation of the tracing and the decisions made based on the result.

Patients with myocardial ischaemia are commonly seen in the accident and emergency department. McCallion *et al.* have shown that mistakes in analysing ECGs in these departments are common, although fortunately rarely lead to problems with management. They recommend that all ECGs taken in a department should be audited, and that training programmes to guide interpretation of ECGs should be created for new staff.[13]

Assessment of quality of care needs to be a continuous process. In suspected angina it could centre around an outcome measure such as the proportion achieving complete relief of symptoms. Units should be encouraged to keep a database of referrals for further investigation such as angiography. The British Cardiac Society could be instrumental in developing the necessary software to achieve national standardisation.

The specialist cardiac centre

The facilities and clinical procedures of a specialist cardiac centre are open to audit in the same way as those of the district general hospital. A visit by an outside team unconnected with the area near the hospital might provide useful guidance on the management of the facilities. The accessibility of a centre's services should be charted, and waiting times for coronary angiography, coronary angioplasty and coronary artery surgery should be made available to those working in the centre and to those referring patients from outside on a regular basis. The appropriateness of referral for further investigations could be analysed, and a league table of the number of referrals related to population served should be fed back to the district hospitals. Chapter 12 shows that referral rates can vary markedly,[14] and questions can be formulated to ascertain why these differences occur. Another useful measure would be the ratio of normal to abnormal coronary angiograms; if this is too high, more emphasis might have to be placed on the development of clinical skills and interpretation on the results of non-invasive investigations. Purchasers and those referring patients for further investigation should also have access to rates of complications related to cardiac catheterisation, angioplasty and coronary artery surgery. This information, collected routinely, should enable each centre to audit its complications and respond to problems, and will allow those referring patients for this investigation to give them a valid estimate of risks associated with the procedure.[15] Chapter 11 by Professor de Bono shows how this process of monitoring can be accomplished by entering a minimum amount of data on to a database; in addition to providing information about numbers of procedures performed, this monitoring can reveal the proportion of patients going on to angioplasty or surgery. This proportion, as well as those with normal coronary arteries mentioned above, could provide a continuing process of feedback to physicians as to the appropriateness of referral. Adverse events associated with coronary artery surgery must be corrected for the case-mix of patients undergoing operation. Models have been developed to allow for this.[16] Information concerning angioplasty on a national level is already available through the British Cardiovascular Intervention Group.[17]

Conclusions

The chapters in this book show that the activities involved in managing the patient with suspected angina throw up many possibilities for audit. Audit of the structure of facilities, as has been performed recently by the British Cardiac Society, will undoubtedly reveal deficiencies in staff and equipment. A regular review of these at regional level may help the individual cardiologist to create improvements. This could lead to a formal accreditation process with the possibility of withdrawal of approval by the profession for the evaluation of certain categories of patients if facilities are inadequate. It is increasingly likely that purchasers will require some such specification of the services that can be provided.

Assessing the use of these facilities will also reveal variations in practice. Cardiologists need to provide guidelines for their colleagues on the appropriate use of these resources (see Chapter 15). This analysis would be enhanced if each centre had the technology to collect and store recommended data sets (Chapters 14 and 15). Clinical audit is a necessary part of postgraduate and continuing medical education, and has the potential to improve the standard of care received by patients with ischaemic heart disease.[18]

References

1. Donabedian A. Evaluating the quality of medical care. Part 3. *Milbank Memorial Fund Quarterly* 1966; **2**: 166–203.
2. Heath DA, Kendall MJ, Hoffenberg R, Wade OL, Bishop JM. Medical audits. *Journal of the Royal College of Physicians of London* 1980; **14**: 200–1.
3. Heath DA. Medical audit in general medicine. *Journal of the Royal College of Physicians of London* 1981; **15**: 197–9.
4. *Medical audit: what, why and how?* First report. London: Royal College of Physicians, 1989.
5. *Medical audit.* Second report. London: Royal College of Physicians, 1993.

6. Report of the Standing Committee on Postgraduate Medical Education. *Medical audit: the educational implications*, 1989.
7. Shaw CD, Costain DW. Guidelines for medical audit: seven principles. *British Medical Journal* 1989; **299**: 498–9.
8. Gabbay J, McNicol MC, Spilby J, Davies SC, Layton AJ. What did audit achieve? Lessons from preliminary evaluation of a year's medical audit. *British Medical Journal* 1990; **301**: 526–9.
9. Mitchell MW, Fowkes FGR. Audit reviewed: does feedback on performance change clinical behaviour? *Journal of the Royal College of Physicians of London* 1985; **19**: 251–4.
10. McIntyre N, Popper K. The critical attitude in medicine: the need for new ethics. *British Medical Journal* 1983; **287**: 1919–23.
11. Lehr H, Strosberg M. Quality improvement in health care: is the patient still left out? *Quality Review Bulletin* 1991; **17**: 326–9.
12. Joint Cardiology Committee of the Royal College of Physicians of London and the Royal College of Surgeons of England. Provision of services for the diagnosis and treatment of heart disease. *British Heart Journal* 1992; **67**: 106–16.
13. McCallion WA, Templeton PA, McKinney LA, Higginson JD. Missed myocardial ischaemia in the accident and emergency department: ECG a need for audit? *Archives of Emergency Medicine* 1991; **8**: 102–7.
14. Gray D, Hampton JR, Bernstein SJ, Kosecoff J, Brook RH. Audit of coronary angiography and bypass surgery. *Lancet* 1990; **335**: 1317–20.
15. Morton BC, Beanlands DS. Complications of cardiac catheterisation: one centre's experience. *Canadian Medical Association Journal* 1984; **131**: 889–92.
16. Parsonnet V, Dean D, Bernstein AD. A method of uniform stratification of risk for evaluating the results of surgery in acquired adult heart disease. *Circulation* 1989; **79**(suppl. I): I-3–I-12.
17. Hubner PJB. Cardiac interventional procedures in the United Kingdom during 1988. *British Heart Journal* 1990; **64**: 36–7.
18. White CW, Albanese MA, Brown DD, Caplan RN. The effectiveness of continuing medical education in changing the behaviour of physicians caring for patients with acute myocardial infarction. *Annals of Internal Medicine* 1985; **102**: 686–92.

14 | Minimum data sets for angina: a necessary basis for audit

John Birkhead

Consultant Physician, Northampton General Hospital

The government White Paper provided, for the first time, an obligation to develop clinical audit in a sytematic way.[1] Working Paper 6 states: 'the government attaches great importance to the development of a comprehensive system of medical audit . . .'. Clinical audit is clearly defined in the working paper: 'The systematic, critical analysis of the quality of medical care, including the procedures used for diagnosis and treatment'. The use of the works 'comprehensive' and 'systematic' gives some indication of the form in which the government considers that clinical audit should now be practised.

Following the Körner report,[2] there has been a substantial and long overdue improvement in the quality of management data collected within the NHS. Previous data collection was criticised in the Körner report as inaccurate, outdated, irrelevant and fragmentary. Some of these criticisms can now be directed at the present development of audit. The fragmentary nature of data collection, where data collected in one hospital are not comparable with those from another, is one problem amongst the many that need to be addressed.

The requirement for comprehensive audit outlined in the White Paper stresses the need to move from the *ad hoc* and fragmented to a more systematic audit. The emphasis must move away from single 'snapshot' audit and towards a continuous examination of aspects of practice in important areas where change might bring about benefit within a fairly short time scale. Within the area of ischaemic heart disease, for example, stable angina pectoris or aspects of the quality of management of acute myocardial infarction might usefully be examined. In both these areas there are wide variations of practice which have a considerable impact both on costs and patient benefits. Although the single 'snapshot' may be useful in establishing what is current practice, audit becomes more valuable when practised as a continuous, cyclical activity.

Completing the audit cycle invites comparison of data collected in one period with those collected in a later period after changes have been introduced. Collection of data that are comparable is essential, not only to evaluate improvement with time but also to allow comparison between hospitals. The provision of agreed data sets allowing (confidential) comparisons between centres may prove to be a valuable audit tool apart from other uses which are discussed below.

Some of the reluctance of the medical profession to become involved in clinical audit has resulted from a suspicion of the quality of data collected within the health service. There remains a suspicion that data collection is not always reliable and is all too often in the hands of junior clerical staff with little motivation and little understanding of the data being collected. The development of effective information technology in the NHS following the Körner recommendations was not straightforward; expensive mistakes were made. These highlighted the difficulties of effective and reliable data gathering, and contributed to anxieties amongst clinicians that clinical audit, needing similar tools, was not going to be easy. It is unfortunate that clinical audit, mainly concerned with process and outcome, and organisational audit have until now developed separately, as they have much in common in seeking to establish the most effective form of clinical care for the resources available. Only since the NHS and Community Care Act 1990 made audit an obligation have more resources been available to develop clinical audit. It is important that resources for the development of clinical audit are now properly directed. In particular the clear need for specialty based audit must be recognised.

Setting standards

Standard setting is an integral part of the audit cycle. As yet there is no consensus as to how standards shall be determined. This has recently been reviewed by Hampton and three possibilities proposed:[3]

- A standard defined by a national committee
- Standards derived from published scientific work
- Local ratings of criteria against which local performance could be compared.

How this might work in practice needs further consideration. Clinical trials of thrombolysis[4-6] have determined that thrombolytic therapy is beneficial when used in the early stages of acute myocardial infarction, and the use of aspirin and thrombolytic therapy has now become established practice. What proportion of patients who are expected to benefit receive thrombolysis, and how shall an acceptable rate of thrombolysis be determined? A recent audit of six district hospitals in England showed that a range of 50–67% of patients with definite myocardial infarction received thrombolysis within 24 hours of the onset of symptoms (data on file), whilst another smaller study reported a thrombolysis rate of 87%.[7] An unexpectedly wide difference in the use of contraindications to thrombolysis has also been demonstrated between hospitals,[8] suggesting that there is a wide degree of diagnostic uncertainty in diagnosing acute myocardial infarction. The 'door to needle time' for patients with definite myocardial infarction in an audit of 21 hospitals performed in 1992–3 varies by a factor of 6.7 (data on file). Thus there appears to be a wide range of practice, and in many hospitals no data may exist on times to thrombolytic therapy; where it does exist there may be no knowledge as to how the local performance compares with that of other hospitals.

It is tempting to speculate that only the results of more impressive thrombolysis studies are submitted for publication. If this is the case, then the use of published data for standard setting may be unwise.

A further problem with standards established from such studies is that they may be perceived to be threatening, and may discourage local audit.

However, the use of data derived from audit studies might be an effective and non threatening way to encourage improvement of local standards. An anonymous comparison of local standards with what is being achieved in a national audit might provide the stimulus to improvement without the need for a formal statement of standards of good practice. There may be medico-legal implications from setting rigid standards, and it may be better for improvement to follow awareness of what *can* be done rather than what *should* be done. Thus a fourth proposal should be added to those made above, that local performance should be compared with nationally audited performance. This lies closest to the second proposal which suggests that local results can be compared with published work. However there is a difference in that with the new proposal comparison is not only with the best, as published work tends to be, but with all levels of performance. An *anonymous* analysis of performance can be made available to all contributors with only their own rating being identifiable. This approach will have attractions to district cardiologists; the caveat is that they will have to cooperate with the audit. The implication is that data collected in each hospital will have to be in identical form. The development of agreed minimum data sets is thus a prerequisite to this form of audit.

Specialty based audit within cardiology

Specialty based audit permits and encourages development of agreed standards of clinical practice within a specialty. This is important in cardiology in which many practitioners work single-handed.[9] It will provide a yardstick with which a cardiologist may compare the performance of his or her unit with that of others. District based cardiologists have to share the acute cardiological workload with their colleagues who have principal interests in other specialties, including those who have a special interest in the care of the elderly. Inevitably practice and standards will vary both within hospitals and between hospitals. Examples of this include variation in referral rates for angiography, variation in rates at which angiography leads to angioplasty or coronary artery bypass surgery, and the very substantial variation in times to thrombolysis and the utilisation of thrombolysis which exists between hospitals. The need for audit in these circumstances is self-evident. The demonstration that standards within a hospital lag behind the national mean will be a potent tool in the hands of the cardiologist wishing to promote change within a hospital. The use of thrombolytic therapy within an accident and emergency department may be encouraged by the knowledge of the improvements that this has achieved elsewhere; the lack of such information makes the case for change that much harder to establish. The introduction of a policy of thrombolysis within an accident and emergency department may have revenue consequences, such as the employment of a triage nurse. Hard facts about potential benefits are important when competing for scarce resources.

There are increasing demands for evidence that medical care provided is of high quality. This is expected by patients, their general practitioners and by district health authorities. The contracting process will depend closely on providers being able to reach targets that will be set not only by managers but also by clinicians. Commissioners are now charged with a duty to provide appropriate care; with the development of contracts they will be expected to account for outcomes within their district. For example, they may be asked to justify low referral rates from their district for coronary angiography, or prolonged door to needle times for thrombolytic therapy. Such data can only be provided with the help of clinicians and, indeed, if collected without the support and agreement of clinicians, the response to any conclusions drawn from such data will be predictably derisory. If clinicians think that information upon which resource decisions are made is not satisfactory or relevant, it is up to them to remedy this. In the absence of good comparative data, managers may have to fall back on intuition or published data, neither of which may be realistic or appropriate to local circumstances.

It should also be recognised that good data form an essential tool with which to negotiate improved services provided by tertiary referral centres. Examination of changes in the pattern of provision of care for patients with angina, the waiting times for angiography, and for coronary revascularisation procedures will require careful data collection over a period of time. The end results may be very valuable,[10,11] and will not be available from any other source.

Experience with comparative audit in surgery

Surgeons have made more progress than others in the development of comparative audit. This may be because surgical practice has more clearly defined outcomes and more clearly defined patient episodes than in typical medical practice. Their experience highlights both the strengths and weaknesses of the use of minimum data sets. It is instructive to examine the 'basic minimum data set' presented in *Guidelines for surgical audit by computer.*[12] This minimum data set contains 59 data fields pertaining to a surgical admission, of which about 20% are patient identifiers, and thus of no relevance to audit. This data set incorporates information that has to satisfy the needs not only of audit but also of summary writing, resource management and Körner statistics. The risks of attempting to satisfy too many interests are clearly illustrated. A summary for the clinical record or for a general practitioner will not need to include the same data as might need to be collected for audit of a particular aspect of surgical practice. Whilst complex data sets of this nature are now much easier to handle with modern microcomputers, which can communicate directly with the hospital patient administration system, the data still have to be entered for the first time into an electronic medium, and it is likely that this task will fall on junior staff. It is an essential principle of information systems that data items should only be collected once, rather than being entered repeatedly by different staff. Only in this way can junior staff and hard-pressed secretaries cope. If data collection and data entry are delegated to audit personnel, the control of data collection can too easily move from the responsibility of the clinician to the administration, with attendant risks to autonomy. Furthermore flexibility, which is an essential part of clinical audit, is lost as the complexity and the demands of the data set increase.

The Royal College of Surgeons now provides a confidential comparative audit service. Contributors have access to pooled data which allows them to put their own data into perspective. The provision of a confidential service of this nature seems to be valuable, and has replaced the previous individual surgical data collection and analysis programmes from which the extraction of comparative data was not easy.

Development of minimum data sets

Minimum data sets allow collection of data in a constant format for any purpose, such as discharge summaries or management data, or in this context, audit. The use of agreed data sets is essential for comparative audit. Experience from the Royal College of Surgeons has shown that design of data sets is not easy where the interests of more than one group are involved. Minimum data sets will always be a compromise between what is desirable and what is feasible. Great care has to be taken in the design stage that data sets remain minimal in content, and that competing interests do not produce an unwieldy compromise.

In developing a minimum data set the following considerations should be kept in mind:

1. Clear objectives must be established, preferably by a working group on behalf of all those involved. There will be a primary objective which is the provision of comparative data for audit purposes. The temptation to include more data than the minimum can be overcome by having a member of the junior hospital staff on the working group. The junior doctor will be aware that his peers will be responsible for data collection and entry, and will act as a suitable filter.
2. Definition of terms. Comparison of like with like is essential. Clinical definitions must be agreed, especially those relating to diagnostic categories. The use of the Read codes will permit consistency in this area. The end-points or outcomes to be examined in the audit must also be agreed in advance.
3. For audit of all but the smallest nature, data collection methods will involve transfer of written data into some form of electronic

medium. The pitfalls of this area of audit should be considered, and time spent refining data collection methods will be well spent. With prospective audit some, if not all, of the data will be collected by junior staff. Motivation may not be complete, and with continuous data collection the impact of annual leave and locum staff on data collection must not be ignored. When collecting data for acute myocardial infarction, all inpatient data can be entered in one place, usually the CCU, but if more prolonged audit of performance in the recovery phase is required, data will have to be collected from other sites such as the outpatient department. The method for continuous data collection in these circumstances has to be reliable, and it is here that an audit assistant may be useful.

4. The quality of data collected for audit should be as high as that collected for any research study. Although incomplete data may have to be accepted in clinical audit, it is to be deprecated. If data collected is found to be incomplete, this may be an indication that the data requested is unreasonably difficult to collect and that the compromise between the desirable and the feasible has failed. The considerations of sample size apply to audit as much as they do to research.

5. Where there is an intention to perform an audit study in many centres, a pilot study is recommended to iron out details that cannot be predicted even with the most careful planning.

6. Cooperation in comparative audit should be voluntary. Data collected unwillingly is unlikely to be of high quality. The benefits of collaboration should be made clear. Motivation of staff for audit is fairly easy in the short term, but very much harder in the longer term. There are no rewards for those collecting data for audit, and although the consultant may be an enthusiast for audit, it does not follow that his junior staff will share his enthusiasm. It is worthwhile taking time to explain to staff involved in data collection what they are doing and why. They should be reassured that data collected is not for the purpose of criticism of those collecting it, but helps to improve the effectiveness of the service.

7. Confidentiality is an important requirement in comparative audit; in developing minimal data sets the ultimate users of the data should be carefully considered. Whilst confidentiality of the individual can be protected by the data collected being made anonymous, each hospital will also wish to remain anonymous; collaboration may depend on this being assured. A secondary question relating to confidentiality is: to whom will the data be made available and in what form? Hospital managers have a legitimate interest in the results of audit, and consideration needs to be given to how their needs are to be met.

Minimum data sets in angina pectoris

It would be possible to produce a comprehensive data set for angina pectoris but it is unlikely that there would be any need to use more than part of a set in clinical practice. The compromise between desirability and what is realistic must be emphasised. The time scale over which angina pectoris may be audited, may be months or years. Long-term audit needs discipline and organisation in order to achieve data of consistently high quality. Suggested data items are listed on pages 151–2. From these, audits can focus on, for example, the topics listed on pages 152–4.

Conclusion

Minimum data sets are an essential ingredient of the audit process. Data collection for audit must proceed alongside data collection for other purposes, but the competing requirements must not jeopardise the performance of audit. Collection of specified data sets permits comparisons between hospitals, but further advances in allowing for case mix and comorbidity need to be made. The availability of anonymous data from a number of hospitals with which local performance may be compared is likely to be an effective and non-threatening means of establishing standards. Although audit and quality assurance are closely related, there is a difference between the needs of audit and quality assurance; it is important that the requirements of quality assurance do not make audit inflexible. Minimum data sets permit comparisons between hospitals.

References

1. Secretaries of State for Health, Wales, Northern Ireland and Scotland. National Health Service Working Paper. 6 *Medical audit*. London: HMSO, 1989.
2. Steering Group on Health Services Information. *Report on the collection and use of information about hospital clinical activity in the National Health Service.* London: HMSO, 1982.
3. Hampton JR. Problems with audit of coronary surgery and angioplasty. *Hospital Update* 1992; **18:** 23–6.
4. GISSI. Long-term effects of intravenous thrombolysis in acute myocardial infarction: final report of the GISSI study. *Lancet* 1987; **i:** 871–4.
5. Wilcox RG, von der Lippe G, Olsson CG, Jensen G, Skene AM, Hampton JR. Trial of tissue plasminogen activator for mortality reduction in acute myocardial infarction. *Lancet* 1989; **ii:** 525–30.
6. ISIS-2 (Second International Study of Infarct Survival) Collaborative

Group. A multicentre, randomised trial of intravenous streptokinase and aspirin in acute myocardial infarction. *Lancet* 1988; **ii:** 349–60.

7. Umachandran V, Ranjadayalan K, Timmis AD. Impact of thrombolytic treatment on morbidity and mortality from acute myocardial infarction in clinical practice. *British Heart Journal* 1991; **66:** 92.

8. Birkhead JS, Chamberlain DA, Griffiths BE, Mary Heber, Smyllie HC, Thomas RD. Factors influencing the use of thrombolytic therapy in six district general hospitals. *British Heart Journal* 1992; **68:** 111.

9. Chamberlain D, Pentecost B, Reval J *et al.* Staffing in cardiology in the United Kingdom 1990. Sixth biennial survey, with data on facilities in cardiology in England and Wales. *British Heart Journal* 1991; **66:** 395–404.

10. MacRae CA, Marber MS, Joy M. Need for invasive cardiological assessment and intervention: a ten-year review. *British Heart Journal* 1992; **67:** 200–3.

11. Marber MS, MacRae CA, Joy M. Delay to invasive investigation and revascularisation for coronary heart disease in South West Thames Region: a two tier system?*British Medical Journal* 1991; **302:** 1189–91.

12. Royal College of Surgeons of England. *Guidelines for surgical audit by computer.* London: RCS, 1991.

15 | Investigation and management of stable angina: a summary

David de Bono and Anthony Hopkins
for a Working Party* of the Joint Audit Committee of the British Cardiac Society and the Royal College of Physicians of London

---

Angina is a common symptom in both general and hospital practice. In October 1991 the joint audit committee of the British Cardiac Society and the Royal College of Physicians of London set up a working group to review present practices in the investigation and management of angina and to identify potential audit issues in the care of patients presenting with this complaint. This chapter summarises the discussions and conclusions of the working group.

Cause of angina

Angina is usually the result of partial obstruction of a coronary artery by atheroma. Coronary atheroma is associated with several factors including smoking, a raised plasma cholesterol concentration, high blood pressure, and diabetes (Table 1). It is more common in men, and increases in prevalence and extent with age. Coronary obstruction may develop gradually, or may occur rapidly as a result of thrombosis at the site of an atheromatous plaque in the vessel wall. It is possible for coronary atheroma to exist without causing obstruction and therefore be present without symptoms of angina. In a few patients, angina is due not to coronary artery disease but to aortic stenosis or hypertrophic cardiomyopathy. Angina can be made worse by anaemia or hyperthyroidism.

This summarising chapter is adapted from *Journal of the Royal College of Physicians of London* 1993; **27**: 267–73.

*Members of the joint working party: R Balcon, London; J Birkhead, Northampton; SM Cobbe, Glasgow; S Davies, London; DP de Bono, Leicester; KM Fox, London; DA Gray, Nottingham; JR Hampton, Nottingham; A Hopkins, London (Royal College of Physicians Research Unit); J Inman, Syston (general practitioner); JB Irving, Livingston; M Joy, Chertsey; CR Nyman, Boston; T Treasure, London; R West, Cardiff; P Wilkinson, Ashford; DA Wood, London; R Wray, Eastbourne.

Table 1. Principal factors associated with coronary atheroma.

Smoking

Raised plasma total cholesterol and/or low density lipoprotein concentrations

Low plasma high density lipoprotein concentrations

Hypertension

Diabetes/glucose intolerance

Clinical diagnosis of angina

The most characteristic clinical feature of angina is retrosternal chest pain precipitated by physical or emotional exertion. It is relieved by rest.[1,2] The pain is usually described as burning, squeezing, or pressing. Sometimes the sensation is of breathlessness rather than pain. The discomfort may be experienced alternatively or additionally in the arms, epigastrium, jaw, or back: the relationship to exertion is more characteristic than the precise site. Angina is often worse on effort in cold weather or after food. Pain that is independent of physical activity, or persists for long periods at rest, is rarely angina. Angina is usually relieved by glyceryl trinitrate, but this is not a specific response.

The association between 'typical' anginal symptoms and coronary artery obstruction is stronger in men than in women. The presence of risk markers such as hypercholesterolaemia, hypertension, a history of smoking, or a family history of ischaemic heart disease makes it more likely that a chest pain is anginal in origin. There are no physical signs of angina or coronary atheroma, but patients should be examined for other possible causes of angina such as aortic stenosis and for features of hyperlipidaemia. The discovery of localised chest tenderness often makes possible the positive diagnosis of musculoskeletal chest pain. An accurate *clinical* diagnosis is an essential step in the investigation and management of angina.

Incidence and prevalence of angina

The population *prevalence* (total cases per 100 population) of angina has been estimated at 1.1% of all patients in general practice aged between 30 and 59,[3] and 2.6% of all patients over 30.[4] Estimates of prevalence in middle-aged men based on answers to questionnaires range from 3.6%,[5] 4.3%,[6] to 7.9%.[7] The differences in these estimates can be explained, at least in part, by differences in the age of the study population: angina is more prevalent with increasing age. At all ages, angina is more prevalent in men than women.

The most reliable incidence estimates (new cases per 1,000 population per year), from a study which routinely used exercise testing and a cardiologist interview,[8] are from 0.44/1,000/year (age 31–40) to 2.32/1,000/year (age 61–70) in men, and from 0.08/1,000/year (age 31–40) to 1.01/1,000/year (age 61–70) in women. Applying these results to the UK population gives an estimate of approximately 22,000 new angina cases per year.

In one study, 14% of *new* cases of angina developed complications (myocardial infarction or death) within six months from the time of presentation.[9] In two studies reported in the 1970s, the annual incidence of death or myocardial infarction in patients with *stable* angina ranged from 3% to 4.6%;[10,11] more recent data on unselected populations are not available.

Relation between angina, myocardial infarction and sudden death

Myocardial infarction results from the sudden complete obstruction of a coronary artery, usually by thrombus. The case fatality rate is about 30%, higher in the elderly, and 50% of deaths occur before hospital admission can be effected. Surviving patients often have permanent impairment of left ventricular function. Data from clinical trials in myocardial infarction indicate that about 25% of patients under the age of 70 presenting with myocardial infarction have previously recognised angina;[12] the proportion rises to 50% in older patients. The implication is that in the majority of young infarct patients thrombosis occurs in association with coronary atheroma which has not previously caused sufficient coronary obstruction to lead to angina. On the other hand, patients with symptomatic angina are at an increased risk of infarction compared with the population without symptoms.

Apart from myocardial infarction, sudden death, often apparently associated with exertion, is more common in patients with angina. The mechanism is presumed to be lethal arrhythmia resulting from sudden myocardial ischaemia.

Confirmation of diagnosis and risk stratification

The *resting 12 lead electrocardiogram* is important in diagnosing myocardial infarction, but insensitive in identifying other patients with coronary artery disease. An abnormal 12 lead ECG identifies a patient subgroup with a substantially higher risk of death or myocardial infarction, but a normal resting 12 lead ECG is not uncommon in patients with severe angina.

Exercise testing with electrocardiographic monitoring cannot be regarded *in isolation* as an effective screening test for ischaemic heart disease. This is especially so when it is applied to populations with a low prevalence of ischaemic heart disease in which the proportion of 'false positive' tests will be high.[13] 'False positive' exercise recordings are also more common in women.[14] [The working group were convinced that exercise electrocardiography should only be carried out after careful clinical evaluation, and the results interpreted by trained clinicians.]

The discriminating ability of exercise electrocardiography is enhanced by qualified supervision during the recording. Time to the onset of electrocardiographic changes and/or symptoms, the overall exercise time, the blood pressure response, and the persistence into recovery of the electrocardiographic changes are all important.[15,16]

In addition to its role in the diagnosis of ischaemic heart disease, exercise evaluation has an important role in risk stratification of patients in whom the diagnosis has already been made. This is further discussed below.

Coronary angiography gives a uniquely detailed anatomical record of the coronary arteries and their stenoses. Strictly speaking, it does not diagnose either coronary atheroma (since vessel wall disease may be present when the lumen is normal) or myocardial ischaemia (since it does not give full information about coronary flow). It provides information valuable in risk stratification and it is an essential prelude to interventions such as angioplasty or bypass grafting.

Radionuclide studies, in the form of perfusion scanning with thallium or other radionuclides, are sometimes a useful adjunct to exercise electrocardiography, particularly in patients whose resting electrocardiogram is abnormal.

Risk stratification is important both for choosing therapeutic options and for allocating resources.

Age: the older the patient with ischaemic heart disease, the greater the risk of an 'ischaemic event' and the more likely a fatal outcome. On the other hand, older patients have lower demands of physical exertion and a more stoical approach to symptoms.

Symptoms: Severe symptoms, especially if accompanied by significant lifestyle limitation, tend to indicate poorer prognosis. However, subjective assessment of symptoms is variable, and objectively assessed exercise tolerance is more reliable as a predictor. A good performance on exercise testing is generally associated with a good prognosis.[17,18]

Evidence of myocardial damage in the form of ECG changes or a reduced left ventricular ejection fraction indicates a worse prognosis.

Coronary arteriography: the extent and distribution of coronary arteriographic lesions predict outcome. Patients with left main coronary stenosis or three-vessel coronary disease have a poorer prognosis; patients with angiographically normal vessels or single stenoses have a good prognosis.

An algorithm for the assessment of patients with a clinical diagnosis of angina is shown in Fig. 1. Applying this algorithm on a nationwide basis would require approximately 3,000 exercise tests per million of population per year, and 700–1,000 coronary angiographic studies per million of population per year.[8,19] These figures do not allow for other possible indications for these procedures.

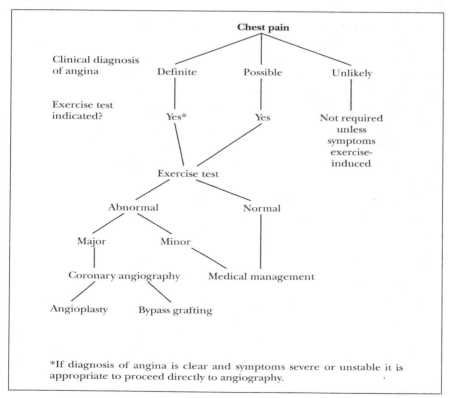

*If diagnosis of angina is clear and symptoms severe or unstable it is appropriate to proceed directly to angiography.

Fig. 1. *Algorithm for assessment of angina.*

Treatment

There are two objectives for treatment: to improve patient survival, and to enhance quality of life.

Mortality rates for 'ischaemic heart disease' in the USA, Scandinavia, and now the UK have been falling over the past few years; there are many possible reasons besides the specific effects of treatment. Aspirin, thrombolytic therapy, and beta-blockade improve survival. Treatment of hypertension, and of patients with heart failure using angiotensin converting enzyme inhibitors, also improves outcome.[20–23]

Coronary bypass grafting has been shown to improve survival in patients with left main coronary artery stenosis, with three-vessel coronary disease, particularly when this is associated with impaired left ventricular function, and in two-vessel coronary disease if one of the vessels involved is the left anterior descending coronary artery.[24] The effects of coronary bypass grafting on survival are greater in severely symptomatic than in mildly symptomatic patients. Coronary angioplasty has not been proven to improve survival.

Medical therapy for angina improves exercise tolerance and quality of life. There are sometimes theoretical and practical reasons for combining two different families of antianginal drugs, for example beta-blockers and calcium antagonists; evidence for an additional effect of adding a third class of drugs is scant.

Many patients with mild to moderate symptoms of angina are currently treated by general practitioners or general physicians. Patients presenting to cardiologists are likely to be those whose symptoms are more severe. Both coronary angioplasty and coronary bypass grafting are effective in relieving symptoms of angina, and both have low operative mortality rates (more than 1% fatal outcome). About a quarter of patients receiving angioplasty will develop restenosis over the next six months, and about one-sixth will have further angioplasty or coronary bypass grafting. Long waiting times for coronary bypass grafting are a relevant factor in choosing angioplasty for some patients.

There are marked variations in rates of coronary angiography,[25] coronary angioplasty, and coronary bypass grafting in different regions and within parts of the same region. These exist despite apparent similarities in selection criteria. There is little doubt that, where facilities are available, patient and doctor preference is for an increasingly interventionist approach. UK operation rates for coronary angioplasty are 148 per million per year and for coronary bypass grafting 220 per million per year. These contrast with USA annual rates of approximately 1,000 per million for each procedure per year.

Current management standards

1. Primary care. General practitioners are the point of presentation for most patients with chest pain. General practice assessment should include:

- Clinical assessment of symptoms, in the light of knowledge of the patient, his family and environment
- Clinical examination to identify other possible causes of chest pain and/or other causes of angina (anaemia, valve disease, etc)
- Assessment of coronary risk factors (family history, smoking, diabetes, hypertension).

Further investigation at general practitioner level might include a 12 lead ECG (either in the practice or via an open access service) and cholesterol/high density lipoprotein cholesterol measurement. (Note: the ECG is not to exclude ischaemic heart disease, but to identify possible high-risk patients.)

Management at general practice level focuses on advice/ explanation, risk factor reduction,[26,27] and medical treatment which would normally include, as appropriate, beta-blockers, calcium antagonists or long-acting nitrate, in addition to glyceryl trinitrate. Low-dose aspirin would also be appropriate in the absence of contraindications.

Referral for assessment is indicated for patients with severe, unstable, or rapidly progressive symptoms, for patients with secondary angina from a remediable cause, or for patients with unacceptable symptoms despite adequate medical therapy. Referral is also indicated where the diagnosis is in doubt, or where a positive diagnosis would have major implications for the patient's livelihood (for example, Heavy Goods Vehicle drivers).

The working party recommends that all newly diagnosed cases of angina in patients under the age of 70 should have access to cardiological referral for further evaluation and, if appropriate, exercise electrocardiography. Treatment with antianginal drugs, if indicated, should *not* be withheld pending such referral. (In this context 'cardiological' referral means referral to a physician with special interest and training in cardiology.) It is not intended that the physician to whom such referral is made should take over continuing care of the patient unless this is specifically requested.

2. Secondary care. Secondary care may be provided by a physician with special interest and training in cardiology, or by a specialist cardiology unit acting in a secondary care role.

Facilities available at a secondary care referral centre should include:

- *Advice* available from a consultant or other specialist
- *Exercise electrocardiography* to confirm the diagnosis and for risk stratification
- *Other non-invasive techniques*, including echocardiography and radionuclide ventriculography and perfusion scanning
- *Access to a wider range of facilities for risk assessment and modification*, such as a lipid clinic
- *Cardiac care unit*, with dedicated beds and monitoring facilities.

Management at secondary care level is essentially an extension of that at primary care level, and will often be a collaborative venture with the primary care team.

Most cases of *acute myocardial infarction* are managed in secondary referral centres, ie district general hospitals.

Referral from secondary to specialist cardiac care is indicated when intervention by angioplasty or bypass surgery is felt to be necessary on the basis of symptom severity or the severity of ischaemia as assessed by non-invasive testing. Referral may also be indicated when the diagnosis is in doubt, particularly in patients with recurrent hospital admissions for atypical symptoms. Where secondary care is provided by a number of physicians, only one of whom has specialist training in cardiology, it is desirable that referrals to a specialist cardiac centre should be channelled through the specialist physician.

A close working relationship between secondary and specialist cardiac care is essential. There is a danger that the interposition of a secondary care step may introduce delay, when speed is of the essence; conversely it is important that specialist cardiac centres should not become congested with cases that could equally well be managed elsewhere.

3. Specialist cardiac care. In addition to providing expert advice, one of the major functions of specialist cardiac referral centres is to perform invasive investigations with a view to possible cardiac intervention. The principal facilities required for this are a catheter laboratory suite, cardiac surgery operating facilities, an intensive care unit, and associated inpatient beds. The extent to which investigative and interventional facilities can be separated has been debated; the risk of diagnostic angiography is small but it

is accepted that angioplasty needs effective surgical back-up. In practice, specialist cardiac centres need to duplicate many of the non-invasive facilities of secondary care centres, and many units function as combined secondary and specialist care centres.

Specialist cardiac centres need to be organised so as to respond rapidly to emergencies; at the same time they must be efficient in dealing with 'routine' cases. They need to set high educational and audit standards.

Basic data sets

Agreement on the amount and nature of essential information which should be recorded about an individual patient and his or her illness constitutes a basic or minimum data set. This information is important as a means of communicating between doctors, for example in the context of a referral letter, and can also be invaluable for audit and research. The suggested data sets listed below for patients presenting with angina should be regarded as minimal, and may need to be expanded in the light of experience.

Basic Data Set (primary care level)

Patient identification: age, gender, ethnic group
Nature and history of present complaint
Relevant past or current medical history, eg asthma, diabetes
Medication
Family history
Smoking history
Occupation
Physical examination
Blood pressure
Any other significant social or medical factors
Working diagnosis
Investigations (optional):   Urinalysis
                            Plasma total + HDL cholesterol
                            Haemoglobin
                            12 lead ECG

Basic Data Set (secondary care level)

As for primary care data set *plus* Urinalysis, Plasma total + HDL
   cholesterol, Haemoglobin, 12 lead ECG.
Exercise electrocardiogram (if appropriate) documented in terms

of protocol used, medication at time of test (if any), duration of exercise, ECG changes (if any), heart rate and blood pressure response and symptoms, reason for stopping test. Results of perfusion scan if available.

Assessment of left ventricular function; clinical, echocardiographic or radionuclide ventriculogram.

Written plan for future investigation and management.

Reason for referral to tertiary centre.

Basic Data Set (specialist care level)

As for secondary care level *plus*:

Documentation of indications for and results of coronary angiography, if performed.

Documentation of indication for and results of PTCA/CABG if performed.

Written plan for future investigation and management, including referral back to secondary and primary care.

Audit points

There is a distinction between audit of the 'process' of medical care, for example waiting times in clinics, and audit of care itself, for example whether appropriate investigations were ordered, performed and recorded. This distinction will be preserved in the following lists. The lists also note possible ways of identifying patients for audit.

1. General practice

Ways of identifying angina patients for audit:

  Age/sex/disease register

  Nitrate prescriptions as marker for diagnosis of ischaemic heart disease

'Process' audit:

  Practice policy/agreed referral policy with local centre?

  Recording of standard data set?

  Referral rate monitored?

  Prescription policy monitored?

Suggested 'targets' for referral waiting times are given in Table 2.

Personal care audit:

  Were appropriate investigations requested?

  Was appropriate advice given to patient?

  Was family screened for risk factors?

  Was referral made? Was it appropriate?

  Is patient being followed up?

Table 2. Target times for secondary referral.

Patients with unstable or crescendo angina	Immediate or within 7 days (depending on clinical picture)
Patients with known angina whose symptom profile is worsening despite medication	7 days to 1 month
Patients with stable angina well controlled on medication	<3 months
Patients with chest pain of uncertain cause, possibly angina	<3 months
Patients with established angina whose lack of confidence is inhibiting a normal lifestyle	<3 months
Patients with probable non-cardiac pain for clarification of diagnosis	<3 months

2. Secondary care centres

Ways of identifying angina patients:
  Outpatient/inpatient diagnostic register
'Process' audit points:
  Agreed referral protocol with local practitioners?
  Priority for urgent referrals?
  Outpatient waiting times?
  Recording of standard data set?
  Exercise electrocardiography utilisation and reporting
  Seniority of doctor seeing patient
  Prescribing policy?
  Referrals monitored?
  Return visits monitored?
  Discharge summaries timely and complete?
  Participation in external audit scheme?
Personal care audit:
  Were appropriate investigations requested?
  Were results recorded?
  Was investigation/treatment plan made and communicated to GP and patient?
  Was follow-up appropriate?
  Was specialist referral made? Was it appropriate?

3. Specialist cardiac centres
Ways of identifying angina patients:
    Outpatient/inpatient diagnostic register
'Process' audit points:
    Agreed referral protocol with secondary centres?
    Incoming referrals monitored?
    Waiting times monitored, priority for urgent referrals?
    Indications for angiography/PTCA/surgery recorded and monitored?
    Results/complications of angiography/PTCA/surgery monitored?
    Participation in external audit schemes?
    Discharge summaries timely and complete?
    Long-term follow-up ensured?
Personal care audit:
    As for secondary care *plus:*
    Indications for invasive investigation recorded?
    Results of invasive investigation recorded and communicated?
    Indications for PTCA/CABG recorded?
    Outcome of PTCA/CABG recorded/communicated?
    Follow-up plans recorded?

Acknowledgements

The working party was set up under the auspices of the Joint Audit Committee for Cardiology of the British Cardiac Society and the Royal College of Physicians of London. This chapter was prepared as a summary of the papers presented to the working party, which have been edited, and from earlier chapters of this book, with the exception of Chapter 9 which was commissioned after the workshop. We are grateful to Dr Robert West and Dr Michael Joy for helpful criticism of the manuscript. D de B is supported by the British Heart Foundation.

References

1. Heberden W. On angina pectoris. *Medical Transactions of the Royal College of Physicians* 1768, tr W Heberden Jr, 1818.
2. Matthews MB. Clinical diagnosis. In Julian DG, ed. *Angina pectoris*, 2nd edn. Edinburgh: Churchill Livingstone, 1985.
3. Research committee, Northern Region Faculty, Royal College of General Practitioners. Study of angina in patients aged 30–59 in general practice. *British Medical Journal* 1982; **285**: 1319–22.
4. Cannon PJ, Cannell PA, Stockley IH, Garner ST, Hampton JR.

Prevalence of angina as assessed by a survey of prescriptions for nitrates. *Lancet* 1988; **1**: 979–81.

5. Reid DD, Brett GZ, Hamilton PJS, Jarrett RJ, Keen H, Rose G. Cardiorespiratory disease and diabetes among middle-aged male civil servants. A study of screening and intervention. *Lancet* 1974; **i**: 469–73.

6. WHO European Collaborative Group. Multifactorial trial in the prevention of coronary heart disease. 1. Recruitment and critical findings. *European Heart Journal* 1980; **1**: 73–80.

7. Shaper AG, Cook DG, Walker M, MacFarlane PW. Prevalence of ischaemic heart disease in middle-aged British men. *British Heart Journal* 1984; **51**: 595–605.

8. Gandhi MM, Lampe F, Wood DA. Incidence of stable angina pectoris. *European Heart Journal* 1992; **13**: 181–9.

9. Duncan B, Fulton M, Morrison SL, *et al.* Prognosis of new and worsening angina pectoris. *British Medical Journal* 1976; **1**: 981–5.

10. Fry J. The natural history of angina in a general practice. *Journal of the Royal College of General Practitioners* 1976; **26**: 643–8.

11. Kannel WB, Feinleib M. Natural history of angina in the Framingham study. Prognosis and survival. *American Journal of Cardiology* 1972; **29**: 154–62.

12. Wilcox RG, Von der Liffe G, Olsson CG, Jensen G, Skene AM, Hampton JR for the Asset Study Group. Trial of tissue plasminogen activator for mortality reduction in acute myocardial infarction. Anglo Scandinavian Study of Early Thrombolysis (ASSET). *Lancet* 1988; **ii**: 525–30.

13. Froelicher VF, Thompson AG, Wolthius A, *et al.* Angiographic abnormalities in asymptomatic aircrewmen with electrocardiographic abnormalities. *American Journal of Cardiology* 1974; **39**: 32–40.

14. Melin JA, Wijns W, VanButsele RJ, *et al.* Alternative diagnostic strategies for coronary artery disease in women. *Circulation* 1985; **71**: 535–42.

15. Detry JMR, Robert A, Luwaert TR, *et al.* Diagnostic value of computerised exercise testing in men without previous myocardial infarction. *European Heart Journal* 1985; **6**: 227–38.

16. Mark DB, Shaw L, Harrell FE, *et al.* Prognostic value of a treadmill exercise score in outpatients with suspected coronary disease. *New England Journal of Medicine* 1991; **325**: 849–53.

17. Gordon DJ, Ekelund LG, Karon JM, *et al.* Predictive value of the exercise test for mortality in North American men. *Circulation* 1986; **74**: 252–60.

18. Weiner DA, Ryan TJ, McCabe CH, *et al.* Prognostic importance of a clinical profile and exercise test in medically treated patients with coronary artery disease. *Journal of the American College of Cardiology* 1984; **3**: 772–9.

19. MacRae CA, Marber MS, Keywood C, Joy M. The need for invasive cardiological assessment and intervention; a ten-year review. *British Heart Journal* 1992; **67**: 200–3.

20. Nyman I, Larsson H, Wallentin L, and research group on instability in coronary disease in south east Sweden. Prevention of serious cardiac

events by low dose aspirin in patients with silent myocardial ischaemia. *Lancet* 1992; **340**: 497–501.

21. Norwegian multicentre study group. Timolol-induced reduction in mortality and reinfarction in patients surviving acute myocardial infarction. *New England Journal of Medicine* 1981; **304**: 801–7.

22. ISIS-2 Collaborative Group. Randomised trial of intravenous streptokinase, oral aspirin, both or neither among 17,187 cases of suspected acute myocardial infarction: ISIS-2. *Lancet* 1988; **ii**: 349–60.

23. Report of the British Hypertension Working Party: Treating mild hypertension. *British Medical Journal* 1989; **298**: 694–8.

24. Joint AHA/ACC Task Force. Guidelines and indications for coronary artery bypass graft surgery. *Journal of the American College of Cardiology* 1991; **17**: 543–89.

25. Gray D, Hampton JR, Bernstein SJ, *et al.* Audit of coronary angiography and bypass surgery. *Lancet* 1990; **335**: 1317–20.

26. Royal College of General Practitioners. Guidelines for the management of hyperlipidaemia in general practice. Occasional Paper No. 55, Royal College of General Practitioners, London, 1992.

27. Rossouw JE, Lewis B, Rifkind BM. The value of lowering cholesterol after myocardial infarction. *New England Journal of Medicine* 1990; **323**: 1112–8.